MARITAL INTIMACY

A Catholic Perspective

Joan Meyer Anzia, M.D.
and
Mary G. Durkin, D.Mn.

LOYOLA UNIVERSITY PRESS
Chicago, Illinois 60657

Marital Intimacy ©1980 by Joan Meyer Anzia and Mary G. Durkin. Second printing 1982.
ISBN 8294-0404-X

All rights reserved. No part of this work may be reproduced or transmitted in any form or by any means, electronic or mechanical, including photocopying and recording, or by any information storage or retrieval system without permission in writing from the publisher.

Contents

Acknowledgments vii

Introduction ix

**Chapter 1
Imagination and Marital Intimacy** 1

**Chapter 2
Falling in Love** 15

**Chapter 3
Settling Down** 29

**Chapter 4
Bottoming Out** 41

**Chapter 5
Beginning Again** 55

Conclusion 71

**Working Papers Prepared for Various
Sessions of the Colloquium** 80

Acknowledgments

Often a colloquium works toward the publication of a scholarly report. In the case of the colloquium on Human Intimacy, the participants realized that the manner in which we studied marital intimacy was much broader than the usual scholarly method of a specific academic discipline. Therefore, we chose to issue a report that reflects our method of study.

Following a meeting of social scientists and theologians at the University of Notre Dame in 1977 (Vatican III: The Work That Needs To Be Done) at which Teresa Sullivan delivered a paper underlining the implications of demographic changes for human intimacy, several participants proposed the formation of an interdisciplinary colloquium on the topic of human intimacy. This volume is basically drawn from meetings of this colloquium over a two-year period. The four meetings during this time were funded by different groups and the roster of participants changed somewhat with each successive meeting (although a number of members were present throughout). At each session several participants presented working papers which provided a starting point for the conversations.

We have attempted to delineate some of the fundamental ideas which evolved during the four sessions and weave them into an outline of a story (the outline itself was suggested by the participants at the fourth session of the colloquium). We have liberally quoted and paraphrased statements from both the papers and the conversations. Needless to say, some of these statements are placed outside of their original context.

Though we are indebted to the colloquium for most of the ideas presented here, this volume does not necessarily reflect the ideas or convictions of any one participant. In other words, we give full credit where it is due, but we accept complete responsibility for the final product.

We are most grateful to Archbishop Joseph Bernardin for his patient and cheerful participation in several of our colloquium sessions, and we thank him for his kind introduction to this volume.

We would also like to thank the Office for Moral and Religious Education and the Center for the Study of Family Development, University of Dayton, and Andrews and McMeel, publishers, for funding of sessions which allowed the colloquium to focus specifically on marital intimacy. The generous hospitality of Father James Roache and the Center for Pastoral Ministry, Chicago, made it possible for us to gather with the group and plan the format for this volume.

Finally, we would like to express our deep appreciation to Rita Troccoli, who graciously volunteered her time to type our report.

Though we followed the traditional practice of the signing of joint authors in alphabetical order, we want to emphasize that this work is a totally integrated joint effort. As the story of the colloquium unfolds, it will be apparent that the interdisciplinary environment contributed to a method that demanded a constant intermingling of ideas. By the time we completed our work on this volume, it was often difficult for either of us to identify who authored some of the specific lines.

Joan Meyer Anzia
Mary G. Durkin

Introduction

In an article in a recent book on sexuality I emphasized the need for the church to devote more attention in the future to the question of the spirituality of human sexuality. In my judgment this book represents an important first step in the development of such a spirituality. I had the opportunity of attending several of the informal and unofficial meetings of theologians and social scientists from which this work has emerged. I found the sessions very interesting and helpful.

Although the two authors, one a psychiatrist and the other a theologian, are writing in their own names, and not for any of the other participants, I believe that they have captured the spirit of the meetings I attended, both in the substantive content of this essay and in the competent professionalism with which it is written. Their work should make an important contribution to the church's effort to support married couples, and at the same time challenge Catholic thinkers and scholars to further explorations on this critically important subject.

Most Reverend Joseph L. Bernardin
Archbishop of Cincinnati

Chapter 1
Imagination and Marital Intimacy

> A good marriage is the ultimate act of the imagination.
> Arthur Mann (to a member of the colloquium)

This volume on imagining marital intimacy has itself an intimate history. It is the fruit of a colloquium between social scientists and theologians. Over a two-year period we met four times, once in Washington, once in Lake Forest, once in Dayton, and once in Chicago. Our conversations were rich, basically expansive, and constructive. This colloquium produced the love story we will be describing in chapters 2 through 5. In this first chapter we would like to share with you the way in which the colloquium arrived at the point of producing the story.

To say we are a colloquium of social scientists and theologians is accurate but not the deepest truth of our conversations with one another. We are really a group of Catholic Christians who gathered to reflect on the human experience of intimacy from the perspective of our faith convictions and values. Since some of us are social scientists and some are theologians, our experiential wisdom about intimacy is enhanced by the literature and insights of these approaches. But the conversation did not have the detachment and objectivity of thoroughgoing academic reports. It was anecdotal, personal, collaborative, cross-disciplinary, with a great deal of personal sharing as well as professional insight. In the end the colloquium turned out to be a group of friendly people exploring a Christian understanding of intimacy.

The conversations were dynamic. Story elicited story, insight built on insight. All the while practical strategies abounded. The colloquium was a combination of the Book of Wisdom, soaring speculation, and the Book of Proverbs, nitty-gritty suggestions. This crowd likes to think big and give advice: a somewhat cantankerous combination.

The discussions managed to be critical without being abrasive. Everybody was open to different insights and perspectives, giving them a generous hearing before questioning them or providing alternative interpretations. The overall impression was of many ideas, some arm in arm, some just standing side by side, and others off in the corner by themselves. But all in the same room. It should be said up front that these four meetings were not kind to the clean distinctions the academy lives by. No one stayed in his or her place. The theologians were into psychological subtleties. The social scientists were into religious interpretation. The people who were not aligned academically were into everything, clarifying issues and terminology and always tying the conversation to the only world we know and so the one we like most to escape from. And everybody had something to say about God. At first the forays into a strange discipline were done apologetically: "Of course, I am not a theologian, psychologist, etc., but . . ." After a while there was less tiptoeing. People just jumped in any old way. The clear rules for what you were permitted to say were hopelessly and delightfully blurred. The conversation, like Topsy, just grew.

There was an explicit agreement among the group to stay away from the "usual issues that cluster around sexual morality."

This screening out of "standard moral issues" was deliberate and nasty. The planners of the colloquium (who will remain nameless) had had their fill of moral issues. It seemed that these issues unduly focused on the right and wrong of

IMAGINATION AND MARITAL INTIMACY

specific acts and heavily concentrated on sex outside marriage. These issues and their stresses were seen as "statistically fringe" to the concerns of many Catholics. When all is said and done, the sociologists said with their printouts in hand, most sex goes on in marriage. Nobody argued. Then it was suggested that perhaps focusing on the meaning of sexual intimacy within marriage instead of the right and wrong of sexual conduct might be a helpful contribution. "Treat the neglected area," they said. Nobody argued a second time. And so the framework for the colloquium was set. A spirituality of marital intimacy would be developed (sexual intimacy being an essential ingredient of marital intimacy).

A final element in the make-up of the colloquium was a concerted effort to muzzle the theologians. As might be guessed and was expected, this was only partly successful. The idea was to let the human experience of intimacy speak through both the life wisdom of the participants and the perspectives of the social sciences before theology moved in. The role of the theologian was to listen and then to reflect, to connect the insights with the tradition, to weave religious meaning from the analyses of the experience. With this approach we hoped that we would not have two parallel perspectives, the social sciences running on track one and theology running on track two with no juncture in sight. The desired outcome was an integrated wisdom, a rich blending of theology and social sciences that would help Christians who wish to understand the important experience of intimacy from a faith perspective. In the theological world much has been written about correlating life and faith. This colloquium was foolhardy enough to try it.

So position papers digested, discussed, and clarified, triggered new thoughts about the experience of intimacy and about the Christian response to it. Finally all the hours of reflection, writing, discussion gave birth to a vision of marriage as a drama—dynamic, never static, always moving ahead, sometimes to the highest peaks and other times through the lowest valleys, but always requiring attention and imagination on the part of the partners.

The emphasis on imagination in marital intimacy was perhaps triggered when one member told us of Arthur Mann's remark quoted at the beginning of this chapter. Or maybe it came from the theologians' explanation of the prophetic imagination challenging Israel to think freely about alternative futures. Or the emphasis could have sprung from Bill McCready's paper on a call for a perversity that celebrates diversity and appreciates spontaneity and surprise in life. But then again it could have come from Jack Shea's call for the religious imagination to work toward an understanding of how "God acts." All we can say with certainty is that we now can't envision anyone making the journey through marriage successfully without an imagination that is capable of dreaming the seemingly impossible.

We agreed that insight does not produce change, that awareness does not produce salvation, that religious knowledge does not produce virtue, and that morality does not ensure growth in love. But we decided that imagination was crucial for engendering movement in the quest for intimacy. The psychiatrists among us discussed right-hemisphere language, which is drawn from images and metaphor and is a language of analogue, of synthesis, and perhaps of symbols; as opposed to left-hemisphere language, which is objective, logical, the speech of analysis and deduction. It was suggested that the right hemisphere possesses a more complete world image and that sensitivity to the language of this hemisphere could only enhance marital life. There are areas of human intimate encounter that are untranslatable into left-hemisphere language; they resonate on other levels of our experience and can sometimes be communicated by poetry, music, images, and stories. The theologians agreed, saying religious images allow us to realize dimensions of which we are unaware.

And so it seems that we need a vision of marriage which will energize us to believe in the possibilities of marriage; to

IMAGINATION AND MARITAL INTIMACY

believe not that I *have* to follow some specific rules to have a good marriage, but rather that I *can* find love and happiness no matter how bad things may seem at a given point in my marriage. In other words, like Israel at the time of the prophets we need to imagine that it is possible that things can be better; we need to imagine a better marriage; we need to be empowered to do the "more" that makes this better marriage possible.

Our vision of marriage, which has its roots in the experience of marriage and the experience of our Catholic Christian tradition, offers not a cross-free present and future, but a hope that encourages us to recognize both the tragic and the transcendent possibilities in marriage. Then we are free to imagine alternatives to the sense of despair which creeps into our marriage with its *inevitable* highs and lows.

Psychiatrists talked of growth and development cycles, sociologists told of cycles in the beginning years of marriage, theologians spoke of death and resurrection themes in religious traditions, married people shared stories of peaks and troughs in their sexual intimacy. And the colloquium found itself zeroing in on the cycles of marital intimacy.

Of course, everyone knows there are cycles in marriage. Who hasn't heard it said, "Every marriage has its ups and downs"? And ever since *Passages* became the explanation for every coping problem experienced by adults, we've all heard something like: "Well, their marriage broke up because he was going through a midlife crisis," or "She was in a Catch-22 bind," or "They were out of synch in their life cycles." And every married person knows there are times when sex is great and then stretches when it is very passable. As John Kotre put it, "While there may be a few Last Suppers in the life of sexual intimacy . . . there are many more trips to McDonald's." At the end of the colloquium we began imagining how the reality of cycles in marriage could be a positive force in the journey of marital intimacy. Ideas came tumbling out. From Jack Shea we heard the process view that the need for intimacy can be understood as an instance of the divine lure to beauty. It is energized by the twin drives of harmony and intensity. An intimate relationship yearns to be a reconciled one, harmoniously integrating the persons involved. Yet this "getting along" can turn deadly if the harmony is a surface achievement which has screened out depth feelings. In this situation the impulse to intimacy may lead toward intensity, living with the inevitable discord in the hope of higher harmony. This understanding of intimacy allows for both intimate peace and intimate conflict.

Bill McCready pointed out that "life gets better if we are committed to a quest" is the theme of many books dealing with "life cycles." Bruno Manno added that, in a general developmental sense, as we journey through the adult years neglected aspects of the self as well as unexpected questions and circumstances force us to undergo periodic times of reflection and reevaluation. The challenge at each of these junctures is to wisely integrate in a maturely responsible way all of one's disparate experiences with the phenomenon of intimacy into a dynamic, living heritage. Our vision is about a quest for beauty that helps married life get better all the time because we learn how to integrate our marital cycles into a dynamic living intimacy.

For some the image of cycles means endless circles piled on top of each other—a constant going back to the beginning, a monotonous repetition of "the same old thing"; and when "the same old thing" is mostly McDonald's, the thought of repetitions is not terribly inspirational. But our vision sees marital intimacy as a lifelong religio-psychosocial-sexual journey that goes through cycles, stretching in an upward spiral, with periodic movement along a plane and less frequent dips downward before moving on toward the goal of genuine intimacy.

At crucial points in the journey we realize that life is getting better all the time, that love is being reborn. Here we can discover the presence of God in the rhythm of human love. The theologians said God language would point to

God's part in our journey. So they repeated the Bible stories about Creation, the Exodus, the Incarnation, Death, and Resurrection, Jesus' relationship with his disciples, and Paul's problems with his new converts; these indicate cycles throughout salvation history. Stories run through the Bible of love freely bestowed by a loving, passionate God who is at first accepted, but then taken for granted and finally rejected by a chosen people; yet the ending is reconciliation and a better understanding of the Gift of Love. Our vision imagines the impossible because of a sense of hope grounded in these stories.

At other critical points in the journey we are painfully aware that we can and do sin. We freely choose not to hope anymore when we encounter obstacles that need to be overcome—for example, discussing with our spouse the problems of our apparent dissimilar sexual rhythms. If we cannot be God with no limits, then we might just as well give up. We lose our ability to imagine an alternative future. We despair. But here again, stories of forgiveness abound in the Bible, and the tradition of grace offers us the promise that radical forgiveness and acceptance have already been given to us as the pure, justifying grace of Jesus. As Davis Tracy observed, using a passage from Ezekiel, "Our hearts of stone are replaced with hearts of flesh" by grace which displaces our constant temptation to get trapped within ourselves. We can risk possible rejection of our advance to our spouse because, despite all indications to the contrary, we know "that reality itself is finally gracious; that the final reality with which we all must deal is neither our own pathetic attempts at self-salvation, nor the tragedy of life in all its masks, nor even the frightening reality of sin in our constant attempts to delude ourselves and others, but rather the hard, unyielding reality of the Pure, Unbounded Love disclosed to us in God's revelation of who God is and who we too finally are in Christ Jesus." We are free to imagine the seemingly impossible because God, who is love, wants us to be lovers.

Someone in the colloquium mentioned that our quest for

sexual intimacy is grounded in human evolution. Recent scientific studies as well as reflections on the Book of Genesis by Pope John Paul II combine to give us a sense of the radical power of our ability to love. We fall in love, it seems, because God planned it that way.

The assumption of such disciplines as comparative primatology, sociobiology, and physical anthropology is that the human species had to develop the capacity for "love" (in the sense of a sustained, sexually motivated relationship between male and female) before it could evolve into *homo sapiens*. The developmental process apparently selected for those genes that inclined the proto-hominid couple to form a "quasi-pair bond" with one another. The main reason for this seems to be that the offspring of such couples were more likely to survive the rigors of growing to maturity—rigors especially difficult for an evolving species—if there was sustained and collaborative protection by both parents. The stronger and more durable the link between the couple, the longer the period of dependency for the offspring. The result was a more elaborate cultural socialization as opposed to a purely instinctual program.

Pair bonding is extremely powerful in some lower species, especially birds. It is rare, however, in higher primates. They may establish a "harem" relationship between a strong male and many females, as in the case of baboons and gorillas, or they may follow a sexual freedom model, as in the case of chimpanzees. The quasi-pair bonding in the human couple (*quasi* because it is not as strongly programmed as in, let us say, quails, and it can be and is broken) is what distinguishes human sexuality from that of the other primates. Much of what is distinctive about human sexuality seems to be linked to re-enforcing the pair bond rather than reproducing the species. A primate species can quite effectively reproduce with both sexes being interested in sex only a few days a year, and with brief, businesslike, and unaffectionate couplings. The virtual readiness of the human species for sex at almost any time, the duration of the coupling, the female orgasm, the affection that seems hard to eliminate, the responsiveness of both male and female to tenderness, the powerful sexual attractiveness of secondary sex characteristics (the female breast, for example), the possibility of face-to-face coupling, perhaps even the lack of hair to enhance pleasurable tactile stimulation, all seem designed to increase the propensity for sustained and powerful relationships. These characteristics appear to be genetically programmed as part of the unusual pair bonding that exists among humans alone of all the higher primates. We are highly sexed creatures so that we may "love," and we had to love to become human. Love as we know it now, of course, is thoroughly human, but it is rooted in propensities that contributed to human evolution.

Pope John Paul II, in his weekly audiences, has reflected on the Book of Genesis. These reflections, published in *L' Osservatore Romano*, concur with the view that it is our sexuality which allows us to recognize the giftedness of creation and to communicate in such a way that we are the only creatures who respond to God's gift. We discover the true meaning of our existence in the experience of the maleness and femaleness of our bodies. The woman discovers the essence of her existence in the masculinity of the male and he, in turn, discovers his essence in the femininity of the female. The Yahwist narrator of the Genesis story, in Gen. 2:25, describes the discovery of the true meaning of human existence in the "original nakedness" of the male and female.

"Original (in the beginning, as referred to by Jesus in Matt. 19:4) nakedness" speaks not only of our prehistory, but also refers to the original state of humankind that is always at the root of human experience. It reveals to us the basic reason for our existence at every stage of human history, which is that, in creating us male and female, God revealed to the man and woman the "nuptial" meaning of the body. This "nuptial" meaning of the body is the capacity for expressing love in which the person becomes a gift and by means of this gift fulfills the very meaning of his being and existence.

"Original nakedness" constitutes the immediate context of the doctrine of the unity of the human being as male and female. Our sexuality, as well as the sexuality of the other, is discovered in this nakedness and reveals the divine image imprinted in our bodies from the beginning. Man and woman constitute two different ways of the human "being a body," the unity of that divine image.

And when we move to the depth of man—male and female—and see through the "eyes of the body," we discover that the exterior perception expressed by physical nakedness has a corresponding interior fullness. Our bodies, from the beginning, through their male and femaleness, enable man and woman to communicate according to the communion of persons willed by God and to discover the gift of love, which was bestowed on us by our very creation. Even though this original experience has undergone changes and distortions in "historical" time, it continues to be a sign of the image of God.

So the writer of the Yahwist narrative and some contemporary scientists agree that the powerful sexual drive allowed us to become human, that is, to become lovers. The quest to rediscover the image of God in our masculinity and femininity is probably not apparent to most lovers, but their behavior grows out of strong genetic inclinations. Like the Yahwist narrator, we participants in the colloquium believe God gave these inclinations to us as a gracious gift. Being in love is a way of discovering the awe and wonder of the mystery of creation and of our own existence.

So the colloquium developed the plot in a love story— focusing on key moments in a marriage—from the bliss and ecstasy of the falling in love of courtship and early marriage, through the settling down of the early years, to the painful bottoming out due to surface harmony, to the beginning again of recapturing the beginnings and moving upward, reborn and renewed. This is a love story for every marriage, not the love story of a TV soap opera or a Harlequin romance, but the story of how two people develop an

IMAGINATION AND MARITAL INTIMACY

intimacy that sustains them, come what may, through the lifetime of their marriage.

It is the story of the key moments in the marriage journey, focusing on the relationship of the partners, because when that is a dynamic force, it unites them against external and unavoidable obstacles. Of course there are other cycles and other relationships in the lives of married people (we have work cycles and relationship cycles with our children, for example); and there are issues other than intimacy which influence the marital relationship (equal rights, male and female roles, to name a few). But just as the colloquium was not ignoring issues of social justice, environmental pollution, the Third World, and other crucial issues facing the modern world when it chose to focus on human intimacy as a concern for study, we are not denying the importance of other issues when we focus our love story on the intimacy relationship of marital partners. This is a basic ingredient of marriage, an ingredient all too often overlooked in religious discussions of marriage.

Our story is a story of the development of sexual intimacy since, as John Kotre points out, "Sex in a marriage is like a rubber band. The strong sexual attraction binds the partners to each other while it allows them to stretch apart—but not fall apart." The sex therapists in our midst continually called for a vision of healthy marital sexual intimacy which would free people from the "should nots" of previous sexual morality and the "shoulds" of the equally rigid prophets of the new sexuality. We found both models lacking a sensitivity to the purpose of romance and to the theme of growth, decline, and rebirth found in the beautiful, erotic love poem, the Song of Songs. Our vision emphasizes that the romance, wonder, and awe of sexual intimacy require a continual willingness to die to shame and to be reborn "naked and not ashamed" (Gen. 2:25). And we believe that each couple should be free to write the sexual scenario that is most appropriate for them. If we keep in mind that we are unpacking the movement of God in human life in our marital intimacy, we need not fear the demonic possibilities of sexual relations.

Our story is set in a social context where marriages last for fifty years and marital partners have twenty or more years together without the demands of childrearing (a situation unheard of until the extension of life in recent technological cultures). Teresa Sullivan's insights on the challenges of prolonged life led us to conclude that the changes in the ambience of human sexual intimacy simply cannot be understood unless we comprehend the overwhelming importance of such challenges. We are faced with the challenge of writing a much longer story than most of our human ancestors ever imagined possible.

Finally, this is a story written from a faith perspective. We write it because we find God's revelation telling us this is what marriage should be like. The vision of life revealed by God in Jesus inspires us to believe that as we seek to responsibly share our identities in marital intimacy, we constantly unravel the God locked within us.

We believe it is possible to write an infinitesimal number of love stories using this plot without ever becoming boring or repetitious. A marriage story that is dull and boring undoubtedly has neglected some aspect of the key moments in the story. We offer our plot to all who are writing—or rewriting—the story of their marriage.

We should add—for those who would think we ignore the fact that some people are incapable of ever commiting themselves to an intimacy relationship even when they are married—that this is a love story for those who are ready and willing to deal with the challenge of intimacy. It is for those who are ready for the "long haul," who will undoubtedly live through many versions of the story in the course of their marriage. One couple might find, as one of our participants claimed, that they go through all the "moments" of a marriage in one day and repeat the story over and over. Others will find they tend to remain in a particular "moment" longer each time they repeat the cycle. Still others will only go

IMAGINATION AND MARITAL INTIMACY

through one cycle in the lifetime of their marriage. But everyone will encounter the inevitability of rhythms in marital intimacy. This approach to capturing the key moments of the rhythm grows out of a commonality of *our* experiences, both personal and as observers of the experiences, professionally and in the lives of those around us. While we recognize that some can never experience intimacy in their marriage, we have consciously chosen to focus on those for whom it is a possibility. "One thing at a time," someone said, and we all agreed.

We also are aware that marital intimacy is not the only possible type of human intimacy. Marital intimacy, though, we feel is paradigmatic. That is, it offers a pattern of intimacy which holds true for all intimacy relationships. The parents in our midst attested to the recurring need for death and resurrection in parenthood, and the children recognized a similar need. The clergy spoke of "falling in love" with a new congregation, but also of the inevitable settling down, bottoming out, and struggling to begin again. We all had experiences of friendships where we had to learn to "waste" time with another before we could begin the complex process of sharing our identities. The colloquium, a hopeful group, intends to address these issues in the future.

One of our number, when trying to explain the colloquium to a friend, finally said, "You had to have been there!" We hope this background will give you the flavor of "having been there," a flavor that gave us renewed confidence in the possibility of marrige, a confidence that our Catholic Christian tradition offers an alternative to both the disease model of sexual intimacy found in many of the "morality" approaches to human sexuality and to the nontragic, nontranscendent model of most contemporary secular treatments. We are confident that the quest for intimacy allows a marriage to continue to be a sacrament in the modern world; that is, it is the way God chooses to use marriage as a sign of divine presence in our midst. Marital intimacy somehow is a sign of the union between Christ and the church (Eph. 5:32).

Chapter 2
Falling in Love

> He gave her a look you could have poured on a waffle.
> Ring Lardner

> Few people dare now to say that two beings have fallen in love because they have looked at each other. Yet it is this way that love begins, and in this way only. The rest is only the rest, and comes afterwards.
> Victor Hugo, *Les Miserables*

We look in the direction of a particularly attractive member of the opposite sex who is in our field of vision. Our eyes lock onto the other's. There is a brief, electric communication of special interest. We may be seeing an old acquaintance in a startling new way. Or we may be seeing someone we've never met before. We are intensely aware of the total attractiveness of this person. He is so sexy, she is so gentle looking, he is so strong, she is so graceful, he is so coordinated, she is so bright. We are jolted by the powerful beauty of the other's maleness or femaleness. It is not just a sexual attraction. It is that, but much more. Something about that person makes us want them, not just for a night in bed, but simply and totally.

We experience a kind of physical arousal we never felt before. Our palms are sweaty, we feel warm and flushed all over. We may be aware of our heart racing; some hidden circuit has driven our nervous system into high gear. The very nerve endings in our skin tingle at a chance physical contact with this person, sending reverberations throughout our bodies. The very thought of this person can suffuse our

FALLING IN LOVE

bodies with sensual joy and a feeling of lightness that we may describe (if we dare) as "walking on air." For a time we seem to be surrounded by a positive energy that lifts us above the mundane concerns of everyday life. We are responding to a tremendously attractive, raw primal force that has taken form in the body of the other. We are falling in love.

We proceed along a continuum of linked experiences: an intense total arousal and the experience of the lover's intrusiveness, an enhanced perception of the loved one, a discovery of one's lovability, a combination of hope and uncertainty (hope that the lover will respond, but fear of possible rejection), and an experience of mutuality and empathy.

The analysis of the colloquium attempts to capture the highlights and common ingredients of falling in love, elements no lover would think at all common. Those who are not in this stage are invited to recall their own previous experiences of falling in love. Or perhaps turn to those around you, the newlyweds and about-to-be-newlyweds in their early twenties, their middle forties, or even those in their sixties. You probably will find them on various points of the continuum.

Even if we are consciously ready to meet someone, we can't predict such an encounter. And sometimes when we least expect or want to fall in love, it happens. It may occur with the force and intensity of a bolt of lightning, or it may creep up on us so that at first we are barely conscious of it. There is an element of will in responding to this initial encounter—we "allow" the reaction to take place. But it seems to be the nature of the attraction that we almost cannot resist it. We experience it as a kind of surprise gift that no one in his or her right mind would turn down. It intrigues us, it delights us, we are strongly tempted to accept the package.

We feel a call, a lure to something outside ourselves that offers us, so it seems, a whole new existence. The chaos and complacency of our former life are shattered. Like Adam and Eve we are offered the gracious gift of Love, where

FALLING IN LOVE

before there was, we now know, nothing. Like the Israelites in Egypt, we are confronted with the possibility of a lover who will take us away from the mundane existence of everyday life. Perhaps this other will, like Yahweh, be a passionate lover who never stops pursuing us. This other is offering us a glimpse of the meaning of life. He or she becomes a sacrament for us, awakening us to the need to move outside of ourselves if we want to experience love. Falling in love is a deeply religious experience. We rediscover God's plan for creation. No wonder it is so wonderful.

We find it difficult to keep our thoughts off this other person. We go over and over in fantasy the first encounter. We recreate the image of our lover in great detail and envision new meetings and what might happen. Our longing for this person is so strong it intrudes most inconveniently into our lives. Our desire has no respect for our career aspirations, our daily routines, our other bodily needs. Once we have "accepted the package," this other becomes an intruder. We think about him or her most of the time.

Our fantasies about our lover when he or she is absent are our way of compensating for the loss and emptiness we feel when the object of our new love is no longer present. The plots of our romantic daydreams center around some indication that the lover is responding to us as we are to him or her. Like participants in religious festivals, we are recapturing the beginnings in the hope of being united with the source of those beginnings, our beloved. We are in a special time, a sacred time, which does not respond to the demands of the profane time of nonromantic existence.

Like the lovers in the Song of Songs, we not only yearn for the lover who is absent:

> In my bed at night I sought him
>   whom my heart loves—
> I sought him but did not find him . . .
>   Have you seen him whom my heart loves? (3:1-3)
>
> I opened to my lover—

> but my lover had departed, gone
> I sought him but I did not find him;
> I called to him but he did not answer me (5:6)

but we eventually discover that he was never really lost since he belongs to us (6:1-3). In our daydreams we always get our wish.

Even our fantasies help us rediscover God's plan. The Song of Songs beautifully expresses love between the sexes. Yet both the synagogue and church see in it the love of Yahweh/Christ for his people/church. It is not hard to imagine our religious predecessors trying to explain the wonder of Yahweh as similar to the wonder of human sexual love, especially when they knew Yahweh created this attraction. Undoubtedly some saga reflected on the wonder of falling in love and was convinced God was like the raw, intense energy he discovered in his love. The Song of Songs, which captures the passion of sexual love, would naturally capture his eye as a way of expressing the passionate relationship established by Yahweh. And Israel continues to dream of recapturing the lover that she knows is hers.

The insistent nature of romantic daydreams is what has led writers through the centuries to describe love as a madness or disease. We sense, they indicate, that it is directing us, and not vice versa; such lack of control obviously can lead to no good. We, on the contrary, find the Song of Songs inviting us to celebrate the lure to the other in romantic fantasies since it sensitizes us to the salvific power of the other, to the giftedness of the other's love, and ultimately to the gift of creation which has allowed us to experience such wonder.

This intrusion of the lover into our lives and our thoughts leads the lover in the Song of Songs to compare love with death since, like death, it pursues its object with intensity and will not stop until it grasps the beloved. Yahweh, the original passionate lover, repeatedly offers his love to us with a passion that intrudes into our very existence. First he offers love to Adam and Eve in the very gift of their crea-

FALLING IN LOVE

tion. Later to the Israelites he offers, "I will be your God and you will be my people." Again, and so dramatically, in becoming the incarnated God-man, Jesus intrudes in such a way that we now have the religious fantasy which assures us that our lover is ours. We are free to reject Yahweh's offer, but he will never forsake us. We can find the revelation of the wonder of creation and its creator in our romantic fantasies just as the Israelites did.

But there is more to romantic love than arousal and intrusion. Many say:

> Love is blind.

and would agree:

> Many a man has fallen in love with a girl in a light so dim he would not have chosen a suit by it.
> Maurice Chevalier

When we are really in love, the other person looks pretty terrific. We may find it difficult to pick out exactly what things make that person so attractive, and our friends and relatives may seem to be seeing someone different from the person we see. It's not just that we are unobservant of our lover's clearly unattractive attributes—we are aware that he picks at his teeth or she bites her nails—we just don't care much about this. We are too busy concentrating on the positive aspects of our beloved. These are so greatly enhanced in our eyes that we have no time for worrying about "minor" deficiencies.

When we are in love, the goodness, beauty, intelligence of our lover are exaggerated. Our perception is somehow altered so we see that person as infinitely more special than everyone else does; her attractiveness and goodness fill our view. We hear it said, "Beauty is in the eye of the beholder," but we know that our beloved has qualities that neither he nor anyone else has discovered. We wonder at the blindness of others to his marvelous attractiveness.

In the past this perception of the loved one has been criticized, maligned, and ridiculed. It has been said that the lover tries to squeeze the beloved into a preconceived, ideal mold that fulfills the lover's own needs. Rather it seems to us that an inner perceptual process in the passion of romantic love encourages us to magnify all the positive characteristics of our beloved. Critics say this is evidence of illusion, is not objective, and is irrational. But we find Yahweh's comment to Gideon in Paddy Chayefsky's play of that name a better explanation. Yahweh has chosen Gideon, the least important member of the weakest clan in Manasseh, to rescue Israel from the Midianites. Gideon asks, "Why me?" Yahweh answers, "Passion has no reason."

Indeed throughout salvation history Yahweh chooses people who seem unattractive and powerless. And Jesus continues this in his selection of followers. Why, we wonder, did Yahweh ever pick the ragged band of nomads and bring them out of Egypt? Why didn't Jesus pick the learned and powerful in Israel? Because the creator of love, a passionate lover, knows no reason when it comes to the beloved. Again our experience of romantic love leads us to the Other who is responsible for its existence.

Only after we are powerfully attracted to our lover are we able to begin to know him. We need the attractiveness of his positive attributes to hold our attention before we can ever hope to begin the task of getting to know him. Just as in faith, we find that love precedes knowledge and is nonrational. And just as the unbeliever cannot deny the existence of faith in the believer, we cannot deny the existence of this tendency for a lover to enhance the qualities of his beloved.

As a result of this tendency to enhance the beloved, we find that lovers begin to have an increased appreciation of their own goodness, a further indication of the wonder of romantic love.

The awareness that another feels we are special and irresistible is very exhilarating. How wonderful to realize that someone thinks that way about us! We see ourselves anew in our lover's eyes. We see the reflection of our unqualified goodness and desirability—and we want to believe it's true. What used to be called disparagingly the narcissism of first love is actually a positive energy, a powerful impetus to put aside (for a while, anyway) the doubts and fears about our attractiveness. When we see our lover's passion directed at us, it is difficult to resist the notion that we really are sexy, lovable human beings.

Most of us arrive at adulthood with at least some doubts about our physical attractiveness and overall lovability. Our strengths and weaknesses and our doubts, in a great part, are determined by the love we received in our early years—to the degree we were special to our parents. In addition, negative parental and familial reactions to a growing child's obvious sexuality and their attitudes about early sex play—as well as negative tones to sexuality in our parents' marriage—can be internalized and converted to a sense of shame that retards our ability to enter into an intimate relationship.

There are also fears that evolve from our observations of our bodies as we reach puberty, and our private conclusions. For example, a woman may be disturbed that one breast is slightly larger than the other and conclude that she is not "normal." She may become very self-conscious about her body and keep her fears secret. She may never realize most women have some asymmetry of breast size.

By the time we reach adulthood, we have received a myriad of messages about the propriety and attractiveness of our bodies and have internalized these. Men may fear they are weak, noncompetitive, indecisive, awkward, too short, or a thousand other negative qualities they think should be hidden from the rest of the world. Women can receive messages that they are plain, ungainly, or badly proportioned. Most of us are very secretive about these doubts and fears because we assume others are not plagued with these deficiencies. This aspect of our personalities, which derives from our feelings of inadequacy and vulnerability, is shame. Shame is the denial, out of fear, of parts of oneself.

When someone falls in love with us, all these fears and doubts are challenged. The lover says to us, "You are special. I find you and your body irresistible. I can't wait to get to know you. I want to touch you and be as close to you as I can." When someone tells us in looks, words, and actions that they can barely keep their hands off us, we begin to suspect that our "defects" may not be quite as important as we thought.

The fact that we begin to feel more positive about our desirability often results in actually enhancing our attractiveness. We may stand taller or wear more seductive clothes or indulge in "grooming" as we never have previously. The positive physical transformation triggered by love has been a popular theme in literature, music, and film: the rather plain, listless girl evolves into a vibrant and seductive woman; the nondescript young man becomes daring and heroic. Although conscious effort is involved in much of this transfiguration, many people contend that the certain aura or radiance possessed by a new lover is clearly part of an unconscious process.

We are transformed by our lover, both physically and in our personalities, much like the primitive hominids were transformed by God's gracious gift of *human* sexuality. Like Moses, the prophets, and the disciples, we find new strength and abilities in the gracious gift of love offered. Peter was transformed from a fisherman to a "fisher of men"; Paul from a persecutor of Jewish Christians to the Apostle of the Gentiles; Mary Magdalene became an example for all who would follow Jesus. Falling in love empowers us to respond to our loved one's positive interpretation of us. We hear our lover telling us, "Be not afraid," just as Yahweh told his people, and we put away (for a while, at least) many of our self-doubts. We "are naked and not ashamed."

When we are in the grip of romantic love, we replay in our daydreams the interactions we've had with our beloved in search of a sign that she's returning our love. We not only

FALLING IN LOVE

want to know if she is interested in us, but we want to know how much she cares. It becomes terribly important to try to find out (by hook or by crook) how she feels. We can't just ask because we'd be risking an awful embarrassment and rejection if we were to discover we'd only imagined her love for us. Most of us sense (though only dimly) that our observations are far from objective in this state, so we constantly question our judgment. At the same time even a hint of a returned smile is enough to encourage us to renew our pursuit. As one colloquium member observed, "Even the *rumor* that someone likes me will set me off into fantasy."

This other person is a mystery to us. We cannot predict or divine her feelings, try as we may. We are intermittently overcome by doubts. Is she just being friendly? Does she smile that way at every guy? Is he this warm and affectionate with the other women he goes out with? We construct elaborate scenarios that might give us some proof that the feelings are mutual; in our daydreams we crave the moment when our lover reveals that her passion for us is equal to ours for her. But in the day-to-day encounters with the loved one, we can't risk revealing our feelings too much. We are desperately afraid of rejection.

Yet the unpredictability of the one we love makes us want her even more. Generations of mothers have counselled daughters in the art of playing hard-to-get to pique a man's interest. If someone places a few obstacles in our path, we have a way of valuing our goal more and trying harder to get it. Fear of rejection by our lover only inflames our passion and makes us cling to the hope that he will love us in return. The mystery of the other which attracts us so powerfully is a paradoxical combination of pervasive uncertainty and persistant hope. Falling in love is like riding a roller coaster—we rarely taste such excitement, but it is frightening as hell.

As we search for a sign of reciprocation of our love, we also experience the need for the other to make us complete. We realize that without her we will be as nothing, but we are forced to admit that the "control" of our own future is no longer centered only in us. It now depends, to a large degree, on the response of the other. Love, for us, is apocalyptic, telling us, as the song from *West Side Story* puts it, "Something's Coming." The strong sexual drive that compels us toward union experiences a counter-pull from our desire for personal survival. We live in a state of "happy" tension as we allow the sexual drive to override the need for personal control, but our courtship days are always lived "on the edge," hoping that our fear of rejection will never become a reality.

Our world is shattered when we fall in love, much like the shattering that often occurred when Jesus addressed the complacency of the religious leaders and people of his time. Jesus' interpersonal style overturned and subverted the world of his listeners, as falling in love overturns and subverts our world. Like the merchant in the parable, we have *found* "new life" in the beloved, but we must *sell* the harmony and isolation of our previous self-centeredness and *buy* into the salvific power of the other.

In Christian theology, salvation always comes from without. When we fall in love, we "experience" the truth of our inability to achieve completeness on our own. Again falling in love points toward a religious truth. At the same time the ultimate trustworthiness of the world found in our theological tradition reminds us that it is safe to *buy* the gracious gift of the other.

Even with this assurance, it is not unusual for us to experience both the delicate advances and hasty retreats of courtship. The careful disguise of our true feelings is all part of the game, an experience not unlike walking a tightrope. On the one hand is the strong drive to get close to the other. On the other is the concerted effort to avoid being made a fool. Falling in love is a risky business because we are also afraid of falling apart.

Elaborate courtship rituals exist in many species. They are particularly well documented in birds. Ethnologists have suggested that the adaptive value of protracted courtship might be an increased likelihood of selecting the best avail-

FALLING IN LOVE

able partner—the healthiest, strongest, the most likely to produce and nourish healthy progeny. Some suggest that it is a way for the male to ensure that the female is not already impregnated. Konrad Lorenz notes that all species in which pair bonding exists have evolved elaborate courtship rituals. (However, not all species that exhibit courtship ritual have pair bonding.) It would appear logical that a species in which male and female remain together for an extended time would have a more careful and prolonged mate-selection process.

Richard Leakey, in describing early hominids, states that it was advantageous for a female to carefully select the male that was most likely to remain with her throughout pregnancy and childbirth. Perhaps the fear of rejection and uncertainty in courtship had considerable adaptive value.

Similarly, the elaborateness and length of human courtship rituals allow us to terminate an obviously mismatched relationship in such a way that the rejected lover has an "easy way out." The initial attraction is so powerful that we often fail to recognize that some love goes unrequited. Sometimes in the midst of the courtship game we find obstacles to continuing the romance (e.g., she's going to school in another state; he's going into a business that will consume so much of his time he'll never be able to be a husband and father). Or we may become aware of a considerable flaw in the one we love (such as heavy drinking). Here, too, the ultimate trustworthiness promised by God allows the disappointed lover to "survive" even the loss of this love. For most, "It is better to have loved and lost than never to have loved." The emotionally healthy disappointed lover eventually (though usually not at the time of rejection) is able to realize that, though the love was real, it was not strong enough to have sustained the lovers through the "long haul" of married life. There is even a giftedness in the breakup of romantic love if it results in the lovers' growth and self-awareness.

Many of us reach a point in a romantic love relationship where we are able to declare mutually that we love each other so much that we're ready for the "long haul" together. We enter marriage with the belief that what we share is more than enough to sustain us. We have reached the point of mutuality and empathy. In spite of all the self-centeredness of our search for identity during teenage years, if all goes well, there comes a time when we are both biologically ready to mate and relatively psychologically prepared for sharing our lives with another person (although in our culture the former arrives before the latter). When we are adolescents, we can fall in love with someone different every few months and make commitments that last all of two weeks. Our teenage love relationships are often high on fantasy and low on tenderness and affection. In order to experience empathy we must have moved in the direction of establishing a sense of wholeness, identity, and a stable personality. When, in young adulthood, we ask ourselves the question, "Who am I?" the answer presents us with other questions: "To whom and what will I commit myself?" and "What will I create?"

Most of us know without being told that our own pleasure in love is entirely dependent on the pleasure we bring to our beloved; the goal of our romantic fantasies is mutuality of passion. As new lovers we instinctively try to sense what the other is feeling. When problems and disagreements arise between us, there is an impetus to resolve them quickly so no rift disturbs our pleasurable closeness. How else would we be able to survive preparations for a wedding, inevitable disappointments in initial sexual experiences, and the myriad differences that need to be worked out in the initial weeks and months of marriage? The causes of the problems and disagreements are not as important to us as the pleasurable closeness we *know* is possible for us. The hopefulness of romantic love assures us that these difficulties will eventually right themselves. Just as we tend to exaggerate the positive qualities of our lover (and downplay the deficiencies), we emphasize the positive aspect of the relationship.

At this point we become conscious of the need for empathy; we try to be good listeners and to "get inside the other's skin" to understand the other. The euphoria or "positive energy" that surrounds falling in love makes it easy for us to be generous. As new lovers we do not have to continually make our love self-sacrificial; our state of happiness is centered on the other. Many a lover has described how he is sensitive, generous, and helpful when in love. He feels not only very close to his beloved, but close to others as well.

The lure of falling in love takes us outside ourselves so startlingly that we discover, as Gail Sheehy puts it, "Intimacy is its own reward." We have committed ourselves to another, put that other's concerns before ours, put our happiness in the "trust" of our beloved, and still feel that we have been enriched. We are excited by seeing her, being with her, talking about her, hearing about him, touching him, being touched by him, thinking about him. And it seems that we never have enough of the other. No wonder they say, "Love is grand."

The grace of falling in love is the tremendous power the other has to help us unravel the God who is locked within us, to draw us out of the solitude of being "alone" and start us on the quest for intimacy in a relationship. And we do this with apparent ease when we have fallen in love. As the Genesis narrator indicates, "It is not good for man to be alone." It *is* good when we and our lover begin to discover our humanity with each other's help.

So we begin marriage, having responded to the grace of the powerful drive of our sexuality, with an enhanced perception of the goodness of our mate, a breaking out of the shame that has inhibited our appreciation of our bodies, a paradoxical perception of the possibilities of our love, and a commitment to search for mutuality and emphathy. For a time we are able to risk ourselves and trust that our beloved will not betray our vulnerability. We begin to answer the question, "To whom shall I commit myself?" because, for a time, we have allowed the gracious gift of our human sexuality to transform the fear and shame that have hidden us from intimacy relationships. We respond to God's love "flooding our hearts" (Romans 5:5). We can believe that the romantic love of falling in love is part of the divine plan that assists us as we respond to the "image of God" imprinted on our bodies and strive to grow to a likeness of God.

The quest for intimacy, even in this initial stage, gives powerful hints about the self-transcendence necessary if we are to be successful in loving the neighbor whom we have chosen as a spouse. The memories of this, the "beginnings" of our marriage have the power to sustain us through many of the difficulties we encounter over the "long haul."

In the colloquium we felt that the negative connotations attached to romantic love rob us of the wonder and awe we experience so keenly at this time. So we are in favor of celebrating the positive contribution romantic love makes to the marital journey. Let's dip back often into this period, bringing with us into the present the energizing force we felt in our early love. Because, as Kevin and Marilyn Ryan observe:

> Whether or not it (marriage) is the last or only adventure left for the middle class, we very much doubt. But adventure it is. Few of us do great things and have the thrill of fame and adulation. We live in the shadows of the great and the famous. But many of us experience the high adventure of loving someone and being loved in return. The thrill of being thrilling to someone else is a peak of our lives. Someone has freely and knowingly chosen us out of the crowd and given us his love. Someone has been ready literally to spend her life on me. What is more ego boosting! What is more enhancing of our self-concepts! To have another human being's heart quicken at the sound of my voice or the touch of my hand! What a satisfying sensation! The only problem is that we damned mortals cannot fly forever. We cannot maintain the peak.

Chapter 3
Settling Down

> Who was ever told that the Cinderella fable was untrue because the sweeping and dishes began only after marriage? Even princes who whisked us off to large Victorian mansions had no idea what hours of removing old plaster or sanding floors would be required. How did we know that babies would lose half of every feeding, leaving us with a wardrobe comprised of blouses with yellow shoulder stains? Where did we learn to pick up roots and move with the company every three years? What evolutionary shift prepared men for abandoning the hunt in the jungle in favor of the assembly line or meeting room? No wonder some disillusionment comes in the first years of marriage—we married for love and affection, not for fixing the leaky faucet!

The intensity of passionate romance fades. We adjust even to mutual infatuation and states of bliss. Life moves along, and the career and the mortgage payment demand that we come down from the peak of romantic love and establish patterns in our relationships which allow for attention to other things. The honeymoon is over.

How is it that something as wonderful as the bliss of romantic love begins to lose its attraction and its intensity? Why do we rather quickly find ourselves walking on solid ground and forgetting the wonder of "walking on air"? Is our attempt to achieve some harmony between the strong pull of our sexual drive and the equally strong pull of our drive for personal survival a sign that our love is no longer a challenge to continue to unravel the mystery of God in our lives? As we cease living "on the edges" in a "happy" tension and move toward a balance in our love relationship, why do we inevitably encounter disillusionment? What can we do during this period of a marriage to keep ourselves attuned to the divine lure to beauty that led to our initial commitment?

Although it is difficult to explain why people fall in love, it is apparent to anyone who has decided to continue the love relationship by marrying that sooner or later some of the glow begins to fade and we must be about the mundane affair of life. We cannot pinpoint exactly when this occurs in a specific relationship, but we do know that at some point, usually within the first year of the cycle, we lovers begin the process of settling down. The inevitability of this settling down might be explained by the fact that humans can only manage situations of high intensity for a limited period. Then we must begin a process of integrating this intensity into our ongoing life plans, or we have to rid ourselves of the intensity by cutting off the source of the attraction entirely. When we settle down in marriage, we choose the former.

Much of what occurs during this period of an initial attempt at harmony will influence the future course of our love relationship, so it is crucial for us to emphasize, as much as possible, the positive aspects of settling down. At the same time we must be aware of the inevitable sacrifices (in terms of loss of passionate love) we make as we simmer down in the intensity of our romance.

The inevitability of settling down is attested to by the struggle for harmony that occurs in all human undertakings. We know of the initial enthusiasm of a newly formed government, of the scientists who make a new discovery, of the pioneers on any new frontier; and we also know how some of that enthusiasm wanes as time goes by.

The Bible is filled with stories of the inevitable settling down of people in their relationship with the divine. Adam and Eve moved from the initial wonder of discovering themselves in the masculinity and femininity of each other— to a familiarity with the garden, which eventually led them

SETTLING DOWN

to the point of temptation. The Israelites quickly forgot the marvel of the God who led them out of captivity as they settled down to the business of making the promised land a powerful nation. The power of the Incarnation was not enough to reveal God's plan. Jesus had to undergo a public ministry before people would be able to hear his message. The fascination and loyalty of the disciples in response to the initial call and miracles of Jesus eventually became tempered by the frustrations and bickerings of traveling companions on the journey through the countrysides. The people of Corinth found it impossible to keep their high enthusiasm after Paul left for other posts. We know from personal experience how our commitment to the vision offered by Jesus wanes after a particularly moving experience that has led us to recommit ourselves. How many retreat and Lenten resolutions, made in a period of high intensity, soon are forgotten in the need for harmony in everyday living?

The settling down in intimacy is most apparent in the direction our psychological and sexual journeys take. Though we often fail to see the relationship between the two (sometimes they seem to us to be moving in different directions), the story of settling down is the story of the religio-psycho-sexual response to the need for harmony in marital intimacy. The colloquium's view of our psycho-sexual adjustments is guided by a religious vision that accepts the inevitability of harmony but never allows us to forget our wonder and awe at how our human sexuality propels us toward a genuine marital intimacy. As we consider the psycho-sexual development in settling down, we realize that our continued hopefulness about this stage of marital intimacy is colored by the vision that tells us that love will survive.

As we all know, a great deal goes on between ourselves and our spouses as we settle into our life together after marriage. We begin to get to know each other in day-to-day living together. Our perceptions of our lover no longer are governed by a cycle of absences full of longing followed by ecstatic reunions. We now have *lots* of time together. We go to bed at night together and wake up with each other in the morning. Numerous discoveries are being made, and experiments are consciously and unconsciously occurring. We are finding out that our physiologies—sexual and otherwise—are very different, often staggeringly so! We may find that our biological clocks are resistant to any synchronization (she's a night person; he has to be in bed by 11:30). We discover that our emotional needs are often at odds. Our fluctuating periods of strength and weakness don't seem to have any rhythm. Occassionally we find ourselves wondering how two such different people fell in love. (Initially, though, this is only asked in amazement, not in frustration.)

The ways in which we deal with these discoveries, the ways in which we manage (or don't manage) solutions to the asymmetry, unevenness, and gaps between us in the first years of marriage are crucial, especially for our sexual intimacy. The patterns and habits that are formed during this time can set the scene for one of two general kinds of sexual relations. We have the possibility of developing a relationship that encourages growth in marital intimacy and attainment of skill in giving and experiencing sexual pleasure, one in which the initial sexual attraction is intensified and strengthened to a bond that can resist the inevitable conflicts of married life. Or we can choose to halfheartedly abandon the quest for sexual satisfaction and closeness with our spouse rather early in the game.

To use a metaphor referred to in the Introduction, the extent to which we are able to find ways to sustain the strong sexual feeling between us and our lover—and create ways to renew it from time to time—will determine the strength of the rubber band that will contain us even under tension.

Most of us expect that learning to cook or dance or play tennis well will require time, practice, and effort, but many of us assume that our sex lives are determined by circumstances outside of ourselves. There is often little recognition

SETTLING DOWN

that sex is largely a matter of learning, and learning mostly through experience. We can fail to see the clear choices we have in the unfolding of our sexual lives. As one couple observed:

> While sex between man and woman may be the most natural of natural acts, it does not just happen. Or, at least, it did not just happen to us. Sex is a learned behavior. Again the dance may be the best analogy. Two people can stumble around the floor and call it dancing; or they can make themselves highly skilled performers.

We would add that positive or negative learning can come from the same experience, depending on how we perceive and act on it. Being naked to each other was a positive experience for Adam and Eve in their original state; but, as the narrator observes, at a later point they perceived their nakedness as shameful and wanted to hide it (Gen. 3:7).

After some time of living together it becomes pretty clear to most of us that, in general, the opportunities for nights of passion and sensuous reveling are not just going to drop in out of nowhere. They require some foresight and vigilant protection from intrusion. In a society that values work so highly, it takes a conscious effort on the part of most of us to put "playing" and "wasting time" with our spouse ahead of "work" on our list of priorities.

Eventually we also find out that we cannot expect our spouse to be able to guess when we want sex, and how we want it to be. One option is silent suffering while we wait for her to know what we want—and an awful lot of resentment. Alternatively, we can learn to cue each other in advance when we want to have a night of lovemaking. An arching of the eyebrows, a pat on the backside in the kitchen, a particularly ardent kiss when the other returns, are all cues that we want the closeness and physical release of lovemaking. Some people find the presence of "signs" such as a heart-shaped pillow on the bed also help to let our spouse know we long for him. Cues to our sexual desires can develop into an art form over the years of marriage—a very private art form appreciated only by us since, although all of the norms and discussions about sex are in the public sphere, our sexual signals are an exclusive kind of communication.

Asking our partner for sex, however, puts us in a position of vulnerability that can be uncomfortable; there is always the chance (however remote) that he might turn us down or respond less than enthusiastically. In order for us to keep on asking, there has to be enough positive reinforcement. If we ask in a manner we feel is almost irresistible, it can be devastating to be refused. Like Yahweh when the Israelites considered offerings to pagan gods, we feel—or make our lover feel, if we are the rejecting person—a certain betrayal.

If we are lucky, we stumble onto a particular positive pattern of lovemaking that is mutually exciting; for example, we may find that seduction in a half-dressed state on the living room couch turns us both on. We then have the choice of replaying that scene again and again with some variations; it can become a "habit" special and unique to us. We can infinitely refine and diversify a seduction scene so it stays good for a lifetime. A seduction "ritual" that has special meaning for us contributes to our sense of our marriage as a good story that we want to end on a positive note. Often the memory of one of these rituals will help call us back from a sense of despair about our relationship.

From the very beginning lovemaking has a pattern of successive stages. There is a stage of invitation, a point of uncertainty whether or not things will go further. There are stages for various zones of the body, the mouth, the breast, the genitals. There is a stage of penetration, of climax, and of afterglow. Each stage has its pleasures and its needs. Each stage has its possible mistakes and disappointments. But for any stage to be good for us it must also be good for our lover; and we learn by experience how to enhance the other's pleasure at each stage. We have to help our lover learn how to bring us pleasure.

Helping our lover learn to give us pleasure becomes more

difficult as we begin to retreat into our shame. If we let her know that something she does to us is so stimulating that it makes us want to abandon ourselves to her, there is the possibility that she will try to bring us out of our hiding. It also gives her a certain power over us that we might not want to let anyone have at this time.

We always have a great need to know how we are doing as lovers. We need a lot of explicit encouragement and support. When we are not succeeding, we need to know why. If we are getting the overall message that we are terrific bed partners, it is easier for us to accept occasional constructive advice. But even with all our planning we are bound to experience times when we have a very different sexual scenario in mind from the one our partner is planning. We might be planning a brief and intense encounter and then on to sleep, while she may be expecting an hour or so of sensual reveling. One has invited the other to dance, but, while he is hearing disco, she is sliding into a slow waltz.

If we are open to one another and are relatively frank about our sexual needs, we may learn that, at a particular time, his needs are stronger than ours. For pleasurable sex to continue, there has to be an adjustment to one another's cycles of strength and weakness. Each must have times of giving and receiving, of being supported and lending support. It takes considerable empathy to understand our lover's needs, when our own (which might be opposite) are so insistent. But the alternative to a compromise is no pleasure at all for either us of—a solution that breeds resentment and martyrdom.

With creative energy we can strengthen the intimate bond between us in the first few years of marriage. We can become very adept lovers. We know the other's erotic triggers far better than any stranger could. After a while we realize that our first attempts at developing a sexual rhythm were far from the ecstasy we had fantasized about in the initial stage of falling in love. But now that we have come to know our lover better, we are free to discover much of the wonder and awe of sexual intercourse.

We also find during this period that we are doing a great deal of "fixing" of our relationship, establishing a certain stability in our marriage based on the intimacy that has been achieved. We learn to know our partners as they really are and feel secure in the realization that we have managed to adjust to many of the challenges of the initial years of marriage. We generally feel quite positive about the adjustment we have made. As the Ryans describe what is happening:

> Our independent self-concepts have grown toward each other. We are like two trees planted side by side which bend together in the same wind and, gnarled by the same winters, reach together for the same sun and sky. We believe we are different now because we have lived together.... Instead of making a decision on the basis of our own preference and convenience, we decide after discussion and accord. The end result of forging and molding is that we are different people than we were. We have changed towards each other, shaping ourselves in new patterns. The content of these patterns has also changed. The self which once swam away the summers, now spends them on the tennis courts; the man who ate in late-night diners and greasy spoons now loves French cuisine; the selves which slept late on weekends and stayed up late on weeknights, now together rise to jog or to have some early morning quiet together.

The continuing challenge of our human sexuality is to reveal to each other the meaning of our existence. Whatever we do during this period of settling down that helps us move toward that goal can be felt as a positive response to the gracious gift of our sexuality. Developing good sexual habits and an aura of security and stability allows us to discover much about the "you" of the other person; this helps us begin to form a stronger communion of persons that reflects the "image of God." The search for harmony during this period can be viewed as our attempt to discover quickly the "mean-

SETTLING DOWN

ing of it all." We are responding to the impetus built into our sexuality.

Unfortunately, in our eagerness, we think we have solved the riddle of life without giving careful consideration to the questions. We are somewhat like the disciples of Jesus; they often felt they understood his message, but usually turned around and acted in a way that indicated they did not. We have only to think of Mark's presentation of their behavior beginning at Caesarea Philippi through the healing of the blind man at Jericho (Mark 8:27 - 10:52). Immediately after Peter acknowledges that Jesus is the Christ (8:29), he tries to desuade the Lord from his vision of messiahship (8:30-33). From then on, each time Jesus tries to explain the true meaning of messiahship (8:31; 9:31; 10:33-34), the disciples either rebuke him (8:31-32) or react in fear or incomprehension. The same holds true for their understanding of discipleship. Their concern for themselves is their response to the challenge of Jesus (9:33-35; 10:23-31, 34-35). The inability of the disciples to understand the right questions eventually begins to have an adverse effect on their whole relationship with Jesus (9:15-23, 38-40; 10:13-16). Their incomprehension eventually leads them to rejection of Jesus.

So it is that for many of us, at some point in the settling down period, sex begins to atrophy. We find ourselves using the same techniques (not as an art form, but as a routine) and also the same excuses. We don't spend much time in seduction and then we wonder, "What's so terrific about this anyway?" Sex becomes an in, out, and roll-over routine where one or both of us begin to feel that the other can "take it or leave it." If we ever take the time to think about it, we find ourselves wondering what happened to the romantic fantasies of our courtship days; but for the most part we tend to reach a point where we don't want to reflect on what is going on.

This facet of settling down is part of all marriages to some degree. We put limits on the extent to which we will be vulnerable to our spouse. At some point we stop taking down the barriers, the inhibitions, and say, "Look, this is as far as I want to go." We choose predictability over playfulness and surprise. We don't *want* our lover to be so close to us all the time. We want our lovemaking to be less personal, so it doesn't demand so much of us.

In falling in love we were willing to invest a lot of time in "wasting" time together; now we decide playtime must come to an end. We want to learn to live around our spouse a bit more, to cut down on this uncomfortable bumping up against each other's feelings. We begin to move apart for the sake of less intensity.

We move toward some stability in our relationship as naturally as we breathe, and we find that harmony means much of our romantic love "has to go." We want to confine the erotic fantasies to particular times of the day in order to get our work done. We want to stick by certain seduction scenes that we "know" will be successful. We want to feel we know our spouse and he knows us.

There is a great comfort in the assumption that we can predict the other's thoughts or actions and we don't have to worry about the unexpected. We don't have to be attractive or mysterious for the other—we can even let ourselves put on some weight! We can breathe a sigh of relief and relax. The confusion, the stress, the excitement, and the endless self-disclosure get to be too much for the best of lovers, and for a time at least, we try to take all the uncertainty out of the relationship and "settle down" to cozy complacency.

In the most negative extreme, unspoken and unmet demands build up and fester. We become sexual martyrs. (One man in a sex therapy clinic stated his case quite clearly: "If she won't be interested in me, I'll be damned if I'll take an interest in her.") When we are not learning to increase our sexual satisfaction, we have no way to refresh our love. This flatness in our sexual lives can lead downward into less frequent and less pleasurable sex. As the surprise that had made lovemaking thrilling disappears (even though we are more adept), we ask the question, "Is this all there is?"

SETTLING DOWN

In establishing harmony we select out what we want to know about our spouse and convince ourselves (and sometimes each other) that "that's it." We have come to know and understand each other completely; we deny that there are parts of our spouse that we don't know about or understand. Both the awe and the fear of the hidden other have been forsaken in the name of predictability and security. Our former fears regarding our lover—the fears of loss of control, of helplessness, of vulnerability—have been eradicated. What was exciting was also fearful and awesome, and too uncomfortable to live with day to day.

When we lose our fear of the other, we also find that we cannot be saved by the other. Theologically, we need the other to be saved. We need our spouse to take us out of ourselves so we can discover the wonder of our God. When we have turned our lover into a known quantity and we no longer experience both wonder and fear in our intimacy, we find that we have lost the sense of mystery in our relationship. It is this mystery which was put there by God to help us discover the divine plan for us. When we don't have to transcend our desire for personal survival to "go out" to our beloved, we also lose a sense of the transcendent love of our God.

Alas, the harmonious mix of our survival drive and our sexual drive begins to become weighed down on the side of personal survival. Even as we reach harmony, the cracks appear in its foundation. It becomes strained and stale almost before it is established. We feel a gnawing resentment that we are being taken for granted. We no longer seduce him; he no longer courts us. We begin to test the relationship as we move away from our previous closeness. The rubber band begins to stretch even further. We discover the meaning of "Familiarity breeds contempt."

Most of us sense this loss of mystery in our relationship, but we do not see how we ourselves have brought it about. We don't recognize that our search for harmony has caused us to turn our lover into an object that fits into our plan of things. The essence of sin is that we make ourselves the center of meaning and try to make everything else fit; we stuff the other into our center with no respect for her otherness. We want to control the other, and we wind up trying to control God's gift of our sexual drive.

Again, the play *Gideon* provides a useful example. In act one we find Gideon, like a romantic lover, going to battle for "God and Gideon," but, like us when we settle down, in act two Gideon goes to battle for "Gideon and God." Our sin at this point consists of giving up our availability, empathy, and vulnerability in favor of a false harmony; we leave out the essentials and render our strong, passionate sex drive unable to lead us to God. Like Adam and Eve, we put ourselves in a position where we can be tempted.

The intensity of our romantic love has lost most of its ardor and we become convinced that this is what life is all about. Our self-deception is not unlike that of Israel during the period of the kingdom, a self-deception which Amos denounces in a sweeping indictment (Amos:3 ff.). A similar indictment of our retreat into our center in the name of the need for harmony is found in this reflection by the Ryans:

> Somewhere in those early years, a sourness crept in. We still had a good deal to talk about, but we also had a good deal of daily business to transact, business about the carburetor and the carpenter and lists of names for the cocktail party and of items for the tax man. Every night before the intimacies, there was a pile of messages to exchange and pieces of paper to get out of the way. In retrospect, it seems we rarely got to the intimacies.

As sourness and brittleness creeps into all areas of our relationship, the silences and resentments grow. A grayness settles in on our marriages and our lives. But God never deserts us; as we walk around in our gray world, we still have the memory tucked away in a corner of our minds of that marvelous experience of falling in love.

Chapter 4
Bottoming Out

We had from the beginning argued and fought. What was new was a lingering sense of discontent that could build to a fight quite rapidly. Both of us had gone, and were going, farther than we had ever planned or dreamed of.

The vague, gnawing, restless discontent that begins to creep into our marriage as months and years of living together pass is generally so insidious that we may be amazed at the enormity of the beast when we are finally confronted with it. How is it that something as good as romantic love disintegrates to a point where we begin to feel our relationship falling apart and we feel rejected? Our search for harmony in the settling down period seems to have resulted in a situation where we find ourselves doing just the opposite of what we had imagined in the period of falling in love. We feel a bit of us is present in this story of a couple who attend a sex therapy clinic:

> A couple in their thirties were asked what had attracted them to each other. He said he was attracted by her because she was pretty, open, natural, and aggressive. He now resented her for being critical, aggressive, and "bitchy." She liked his good looks, responsibility, and intelligence, but became disillusioned when he became childish and dependent. He was depressed and his self-esteem was poor; his body image was one of poor masculinity. She wanted the "Rock of Gilbraltar."

At first we may not be able to lay a finger on what is bothering us, but we feel anxious. We sense a resentment and unsatisfied need within us, but we feel even greater anxiety about the unknown—the dissatisfactions we haven't admitted to ourselves. The question, often not articulated, is, "How can good things go so bad?"

As the pull toward personal survival wins out over our strong drive for sexual intimacy, we find that all negative qualities considered inconsequential during courtship seem to occupy more and more of our attention. It is as if the demonic aspects of our relationship have been in hiding until such time as we are ready to respond to the offer to "eat of the fruit of the forbidden tree." For us the temptation is to embrace shame. We deny the importance of our sexual drive; we hid from ourselves, each other, and the God who has created us "in the image of God." We have reached the stage of bottoming out in our marital journey.

It is hard to believe that there is anything good about this bottoming out period in our love story. Yet, if we remember the divine lure to beauty, we realize that the harmony of settling down, which led to routine and boredom, could not really be what God was pointing us toward when our bodies were imprinted with the divine image. What we had in the settling down period was a false harmony that neglected many important features of the true harmony of genuine intimacy. The discord of this stage can be a stimulus toward a renewed search for genuine intimacy. Though it seems a backward movement in our journey toward intimacy, it can cause a dip back into the wonder and awe of falling in love, which will lead to an upward movement of the spiral.

Again, we find that any human attempt at growth and development eventually encounters a time when darkness is the order of the day. As we struggle to grow, we encounter the possibility of our own sin and it leads us to despair. Adam and Eve had to experience the terror of hiding from God before we could hear the promise of the first covenant. Israel had to be banished to Babylon before it would

BOTTOMING OUT

recognize its failure to be true to Yahweh. Jesus had to die before he could be raised. The disciples felt the shame of denying Jesus, but the only one who was lost was Judas. The people of Corinth experienced much disruption in their religious life, but it led to a new inspirational message from Paul. We cannot deny our own tendency to make ourselves the center of things, and our betrayal of our covenant of love with our spouse. We must move from the darkness to the light, but we can only begin to do that when we acknowledge the darkness. The central task of this stage of the intimacy cycle is that of dying.

Our anxiety during this period causes us to worry; we worry whether our anger and resentment are justified. We wonder if we might have imagined the slights and injuries. Are we too sensitive? Do we want too much from our spouse? Would our complaints look ridiculous if we voiced them to our spouse or to other people? Are my sexual needs normal, or will my spouse think I'm perverse?

We find that we feel guilty about our frustrations; many of us reached adulthood with the idea that "good" husbands and wives didn't have such emotions. Model spouses were not supposed to feel used or thwarted by one another. Anger itself was wrong and sinful, a weakness to be remedied with humility and forbearance. As the Ryans describe their "battle not to battle":

> What was most upsetting to us about our fighting—more than all the time they took up—was that these fights violated our expectations of a good marriage. We were clearly failing. We hadn't known people who fought. We saw our fighting as a clear and definite sign of failure. And we felt as if we were being sucked into a vortex.

We find that we are afraid of losing what we have if we give vent to our feelings. The present situation is highly unsatisfactory—we feel trapped, locked in—but we cling for dear life to the false harmony we find in the established framework of our marriage. At least we know what we are supposed to be doing within that framework. To challenge it might mean letting go of it, and then what? How can we give up that security, rigid though it is? We become closed to the possibilities of growth as we trap ourselves within ourselves, refuse to let go, to believe that things can be any better, to hope for a way out.

There is a clear choice to be made here, though it is almost never made consciously. Either we express the flaws, criticize what we feel is not working in the relationship—or we don't. Which way we go depends on many things: our own self-esteem as individuals, our ability and confidence to put our feelings into words, our attitudes about the appropriateness of quarreling, the magnitude of our anger, the amount of neurotic dependency built into the relationship, and most of all, the amount of trust that has so far developed in the marriage. We must choose either to respond to the loss of the grace of our sexuality or never be able to use it to find our beloved and our God.

If we decide that confronting the problems is too threatening or not "worth the trouble," one of two basic situations will result: the relationship will be ended, probably before conflict becomes inevitable, or we will assume a "holding pattern" in which conflict is continually met with evasive maneuvers.

The first option for a couple, to end the marriage before things get too hot for comfort, leads to the phenomenon of the "friendly" separation, the "amicable" divorce. There are numberless divorced people who say their marriages ended not with a bang, but with a whimper. They claim that they just got bored, and there was nothing else to do but call it quits. Or things were just so bad that the situation "wasn't worth fighting about." They were not happy with the false harmony, but the drive to sexual intimacy with their spouse was not strong enough to move them to change the relationship.

Sometimes it is easier for this to happen if there is little social, familial, and economic pressure for the couple to stay together; the childless working couple with no close extended family can separate without much delay and external disapproval. Children and extended family, as well as certain social and cultural norms, are all part of the bond between us; their presence and vested interest in the marriage may actually keep us together *long enough* for the bottoming out to intensify to the point where we have to acknowledge it. (For example, the family might insist that the couple seek some help in the form of therapy before giving up. Family has a way of demanding explanations that may bring the issues to the surface.)

So too, the belief that our mariage is a covenant relationship keeps us from giving up without considerable effort. When the grace of the "rubber band" of our sexuality is not powerful enough to keep us on our quest for intimacy, and we are a "broken community," we find the command to "love our neighbor" (spouse) reminds us of the God we fail to find in our present union.

If we opt for the "holding pattern" approach, we find we won't let go of the perceptions and rules about marriage that governed our response to the need to find harmony in our intimacy. This holding on tends to perpetuate the overall tone of indecision. The relationship is neither night or day, but stuck in some twilight area.

When our anxiety becomes unbearable, numbness may be punctuated by brief, unsatisfactory quarrels in which issues are only hinted at and nothing is resolved. The cold war path is one of cynical barbs, passive-aggressive sulks, series of brief attacks and hasty retreats, and much silence. We deny that the anger and frustration has anything at all to do with the marriage; we focus it on another issue, perhaps on a disagreement about one of the children or the management of the household or any other problem that's available. (This diversion is well known to all of us; it is widely used by all married couples. A decision about who is to sort laundry can evolve into full-scale nonbattle in which bitter words and insinuations are traded in the guise of concern over socks and underwear.)

When our spouse does something that particularly upsets us, we may opt not to talk to her for a period of time. This carries the advantage of letting her know we are angry and making her guess what is bothering us. Or we may turn the anger in on ourselves and develop recurrent tension headaches or other somatic symptoms. Our spouse appears to be our worst enemy. This observation by the Ryans captures what some of us do during this time:

> If, through nagging or ignoring or ridicule, we come to believe that the mate knows us but finds us wanting, then it is hard to have a favorable view of oneself. Sometimes our spouse is our own worst enemy. Some men are known to make fun of their wives to embarrass them, a social game different from kidding them. There are women who work out their angers by belittling their husbands in the presence of other couples. A friend reported that a couple he had known on the faculty in Chicago finally divorced. They had been married for 20 years and the split came as a shock to many people. But our friend was not surprised. "Mrs. S. said to me on more than one occasion: 'You know Nelson isn't very good in bed!'" Surely Mrs. S. couldn't have been among the surprised when old Nelson finally took up with a younger woman.

To satisfy the emotional and sexual needs that aren't being met, we turn to other people—an affair or special closeness and sharing with a group of members of the same sex. We will have romance in our lives—our sexual drive sees to that—and if we can't have it with our spouse, we will find it elsewhere. The intense sharing of women's groups, either Kaffee Klatching or consciousness raising, is often the result of inability to share with our husbands.

If we have been successful in pretending there is no tension in the marriage, sex may continue; indeed, it may be a way of trying to prove to ourselves that there is still some good feeling between us. (Consider the couple who go for

BOTTOMING OUT

marriage counseling just to satisfy everyone that they "tried to do something about it," and tell the counselor that "sex" is no problem in their relationship.) Intercourse may, in a strange way, become part of the effort to hide the anger and resentment. This is a kind of angry, manipulative sex to artificially create the closeness that no longer exists.

If our resistance to confronting the issues of bottoming out is very strong, we will develop more rigid and uncompromising patterns of behaviors. Our unresolved anger often shows itself in prolonged grudges. This story of a woman in a sex therapy clinic shows how these grudges become more destructive the longer they are held, and also less understandable:

> A middle-aged woman married twenty years said she had never forgiven her husband for getting her pregnant before marriage. She was currently accusing him of hitting her and lying to her.

It was easy for the counselor to understand why she had been angry about her unplanned pregnancy. It was much harder for him to understand why she was still angry after twenty years. Perhaps, like us, she had found something to use as a rationalization, one of a number of "good reasons" for avoiding sex, with no need to feel there was anything lacking in herself. When we engage in similar behavior, is it because we lack the skill to reconcile with our spouse, or are we just afraid to try?

A state of incomplete bottoming out can persist for years, until an event such as the leaving of the youngest child, a midlife career crisis, or a heart attack triggers an explosion so devastating that we end either in divorce or in therapy with years of rage and resentment to unload upon each other. A couple in the latter situation came to a family counselor. Their story, while it seems extreme, shows how long we can live with rage:

Bob and Betty are in their late sixties. They entered therapy after forty-four years of marriage because of a near total breakdown of trust and communication in their relationship. Four months before, Bob confessed to Betty he'd been having an affair for eighteen months with his forty-year-old secretary. Betty was devastated, enraged, depressed, and panicked; her self-esteem shattered. Bob was overwhelmed with guilt, despair, and helpless frustration. Sexually, Bob had become impotent and Betty was unable to meet her own needs, much less Bob's. When their fragile bonds of trust collapsed, open conflict ensued with their sexual and emotional bonds of intimacy collapsing soon after. The result was a severely dysfunctional marriage containing two frightened, angry individuals. Both felt powerless, victimized, and choiceless. Both blamed the other. Reconciliation seemed hopeless and divorce unthinkable.

The background of this tale includes the fact that it was after a coronary bypass that Bob became impotent. Through a shared conspiracy of denial and naivete, they became convinced that his impotence was physical and irreversible. Their marriage became strained and tensions rose. Both felt secretly devalued and cheated. Having never confronted and negotiated the powerful emotional attachment between themselves, they covertly conspired to be silent. Bob's devalued sense of himself drove him to an affair with his secretary. At this time in his life he needed to discover the meaning of his existence, but he and his wife had not developed patterns that would allow him to face the issue.

When our marriage covenant becomes frozen and we are locked in the throes of the battle between trust and mistrust, we are not unlike Israel at the time of Jeremiah. We need to have something happen to make us face up to the fact that our intimacy is almost at an end. Walter Brueggemann describes the need of Israel at this time as a need for a "prophetic imagination" which will bring the hurt to public expression and dismantle the numbness. Only if that need is met will a new reality be able to emerge. Jeremiah's task was

BOTTOMING OUT

to keep alive the ministry of imagination, to keep on conjuring and proposing alternative futures.

If our marriage has bottomed out, our sex has become perfunctory, ridden with unacknowledged tension, and manipulative, or it has ceased altogether. We may continue in this restless state to initiate sex as a kind of desperate attempt to retrieve some positive feeling between us. We look for some spark of the former seduction. However, the caresses and fondlings that are part of sex have a way of tapping into whatever strong feelings are contained within us at the time. When our spouse begins to touch us in an intimate way, which used to say "reveal yourself to me," the anger and resentment can tumble out. In this way even unhappy, empty sex may result in the triggering of conflict. It reminds us that we have lost something very precious, and we are both angry and sad.

The last option opened to us at this stage is to fight. The decision to fight is not one that is planned or made consciously. We do not fight because someone feels it would be good for us. There are all sorts of good reasons for avoiding conflict, and no one in his right mind looks forward to the experience. (Most of us do not even like to think about the worst moments we have shared with each other, after they are over.)

At some point, however, we become aware—a pervasive feeling settles in—that we will have to act on our feelings or there won't be much left between us. At this point we may be avoiding each other as never before. Like Israel we have hidden our heads in the sand for too long. The signals of impending disaster are all around us, and we feel a strong tension to do something about the disharmony in our marital lives.

Herein lies the paradox. We sense that fighting may be the only way to go if we really want to move ahead. It may be the only way we can be faithful to the covenant. It takes a certain courage to break the silence with expressions of anger; it takes strength to face the destructive potential within ourselves and our spouse. We do not enter the fray as confident, purposeful warriors; we are scared to death. Fighting brings fear back into the relationship; the presence of disharmony. In a paradoxical way, the move to conflict is a clear indication of "fidelity in time of trial."

Individual stories indicate that fighting in the bottoming out stage may be extremely explosive and last for weeks or months; for others it is less intense and lasts only a day or two. Many of us can point to one or two major upheavals in our years of marriage; others describe a series of less traumatic ones, occurring every year or two.

In addition to major times of conflict, most of us go through a kind of mini-bottoming out very frequently. The issues—rejection, unsatisfied needs, hurt—are the same; but the dimensions of the feelings are much smaller. For example, if we were home with small children while our husband took a three-day business trip, followed by two late-night working stints, we might begin to feel hurt and rejected. Though our feelings are not of the proportion of a major conflict, our hurt is nonetheless real; this stands in the way of a happy reunion between us. We feel that we must somehow let him know how angry we are before we can experience the joy of return.

In most conflicts both spouses are injured parties and perpetrators of injury. Both have needs that aren't being satisfied. The intensity of our anger overrides our anxiety. The anger is our courage. We speak out, and somehow when we speak of our hurts and bitterness, they become *real* and all the more painful.

The following brief scenario is a reference story with certain essential components. What we actually say in a fight at these times in our marriage varies, but what we usually mean is something like this:

> One of us says, "I am very hurt. I needed things of you that you did not give to me. You picked away at my self-esteem instead of supporting me. You turned your back on me

BOTTOMING OUT

when I needed warmth and closeness. You gave affection to others instead of me, to spite me. I *hate* you for what you have done to me."

As we confront our spouse we think to ourselves, "Have I imagined all this or is it real? How could you, my lover, my spouse, have done these things to me when I trusted you? Am I being paranoid?"

The other replies, "How can you accuse me of hurting you when I have had nothing but the best of intentions? Look at all I've done for you! You are *imagining* things."

"It's not my fault if you're unhappy. I've tried so hard and this is what I get! I wonder why I even try, for God's sake."

"You're asking too much; you want someone better than me. You are the selfish one."

"You may feel you are right, but look at me! I am hurt, too. You really are my worst enemy."

If this is all that is said, our fight simply continues the self-deception. We are blaming each other, not willing to acknowledge our own sinfulness at this point. We are guilty (not doing or feeling what we're supposed to do or feel) at this point; there will be no way out of our bottoming out.

But there is a possible grace in our ability to move beyond this fight and recognize that our spouse is raising questions about our behavior, intentions, and character that are extremely painful. Though we fend them off with denials and counter-accusations (he is the guilty one!), the truth screams at us. His questions become our questions. We look at ourselves in a restless state of growing despair. We flush in our anxiety. Tears come. And we both think:

> Could I manipulate, hurt, use you in the way you say I do? Oh, how terrible it would be if I could have . . . I could not have . . .

I must have. I feel I must have, because the pain in your face is evidence I cannot ignore. Oh, my God.

Our fight, like the "prophetic imagination," has cut through the self-deception and penetrated the dissatisfied coping that has seemed to have no end or resolution. And we grieve. As accusations are traded, the blame shouted, the hurt screamed out, we see what evil we have done to each other. We recognize our sins and the sins of our spouse for what they are. In our voices, our faces, our bodies the pain is very real. We go over our own sinful deeds:

> We are jealous, we are insecure, we are selfish. We manipulate, we use the person we promised to love to our own advantage. We are not the person our spouse thought we were. We have undermined what we thought was the most important part of our lives. We are destructive; we are weak. We can't be trusted again.

We are alienated from ourselves.

And there is no righteous anger for the injured, only equal despair. We cannot trust our spouse; therefore, we must not be worthy of trust. We are alienated from each other.

Together we fear that the hurt between us is beyond repair, the vast gulf between us is beyond forgiveness. We are not good enough for the task. We have gone too far. Together we are overcome by a sinking sensation, a sickening, visceral realization that the relationship may never, ever be the same again.

We are hiding in the garden. We are in exile in Babylon. It is Good Friday. We are the disciples who have run away in fear. We are Corinth accusing Paul and we are Paul hearing these accusations. And we grieve some more.

A language of grief evolves from our language of anger. We cry out for what has been lost and destroyed between us. We remember the joy and pleasure of our original love and the memory brings bitter tears. We weep over our relationship, much as Jesus wept over Jerusalem. It is as painful as

BOTTOMING OUT

death, it is a death, and we mourn like widows and widowers. We cannot sleep well, if at all. Our eyes are hollow. We move through the day, going about our usual tasks with leaden steps. We feel terribly remote from each other; we are alienated from the life that was between us.

Although our lamentations might be kept within the silence of our own thoughts, our children and our close friends are apt to notice that something is not right. The joy has gone out of our life and "the yoke of my sins weighs down on me" (Lam. 1:14). How will we ever get over this pain?

But grief and its agony are testimony that things are not right. So our grief can be an empowering cry. Only those who mourn will be comforted (Matt. 5:4). We must engage this suffering unto death. We must embrace the inscrutable darkness. An embrace of endings permits beginnings.

Yahweh has not deserted us. For in our alienation, we ache for each other.

Chapter 5
Beginning Again

> In the uncertain hour before the morning
> Near the ending of the interminable night
> T.S. Eliot, *Little Gidding*

Each of us is wounded, and we are separate and remote from each other as we have never been before. We have been each other's worst enemy. As we sleep back to back, or in separate beds, or in separate rooms, we find ourselves, in all our numbness, craving the sweet physical closeness that we fear is lost. We have seen the weaknesses, failures, and destructive behavior of our spouse, and for some strange reason, we still find ourselves wanting him in a way that defies common sense. Our spouse has seen our inconsistencies, blunders, and outright meanness; by all rights we should give up any hope that he could still accept us after this revelation. But we find ourselves carefully searching for any clue that he still wants us.

Again we might ask, how is it possible that we should feel this way? Perhaps it is that something has happened in the exchange of angry words, the unveiling of our selfish motives, the forced recognition of our limitations, the breaking of the rules of our relationship. In the wake of destruction, in addition to our grief, we discover a passion for the other that is not extinguished. Its presence may be barely perceptible amid the ruins, but it stands out like a brief flash of sun on the frozen snow of midwinter.

We hadn't planned any reconciliation when we started to fight. In the depths of our anger and despair we don't feel morally or socially obligated to return to romance with our spouse. Indeed, who in their right mind would say we could or should possibly hope to reconcile after all that has happened? At rock bottom, when we think that what has held us together has fallen apart, we discover (to our great surprise) that we're still very much aroused in the presence of the other. How perverse! How bizarre! How unexpected!

There is a powerful, sexual, unreasonable feeling between us that we cannot destroy; it seems to be given. It is so incongruous, it is almost funny. We are under the spell of a very mysterious turn of events when we least expect it. The rediscovery of our sexual passion in "the pits" of our life together is a graced moment.

We are like Adam and Eve tentatively moving into the world beyond the garden with a hope that this time they will be true to the promise of Yahweh. We are like Israel hearing a hint of the possibility she will return to her beloved Jerusalem. We are like Peter running to the tomb to see if the stories are true. We are allowing the grace of our creation to unfold again in our lives.

We are reading "with the eyes of our body" and hoping that we can begin again. The lure to beauty of our sexuality is exerting a pull, not just to hop into bed with each other, but to reestablish a relationship. This initial stage of beginning again is a deeply religious experience. We are still quite free to refuse the grace of this moment, a grace that is both gift and command and that challenges and fulfills all our authentic strivings. As we pause before making a choice, we are reminded of T.S. Eliot's line, again from *Little Gidding*, "Between melting and freezing the soul's sap quivers."

This graced event presents us with a particular invitation. Our bodies, our whole being, are telling us, "It's not too late to start again! Don't give up; you can make her want you again." Of course, we have the power to refuse the invitation that lights our bodies with arousal. We have the option of closing the door on possibility, of hiding our attraction to her from her, but why would we do that when we are also hoping that maybe things can be better? Our openness to

BEGINNING AGAIN

this invitation of our sexual drive is closely related to the firmness of our belief in the goodness of new possibilities. We need to imagine the possibility of a new covenant, of a return from exile, of a resurrection.

For some of us at particular times the passion, anger, and grief of bottoming out are transformed rapidly into the passion of lovemaking. For others, and at other times, the sexual desire is responded to with many small steps in the direction of lovemaking and is interwoven with other dimensions of reconciliation. The resumption of intercourse may be approached with great care.

The dramatic transformation of passion is portrayed over and over again in literature and film. Psychiatrists and others who do marital therapy often report that a couple in the midst of crisis will begin lovemaking again, even as angry words are being exchanged. Couples who have "every reason" to stay apart, not to trust one another, are still experiencing a strong physical attraction to each other. The grace of what is often disparagingly called "unbridled passion" serves to shatter the hopelessness of our despair. We were not meant to be alone.

We know that to follow the desire that is taking hold of us will mean a lot of conscious effort in rebuilding the relationship. We will have to court our spouse all over again. We will have to look inside ourselves to see what needs to be changed. We will have to forgive and be forgiven. We are presented with a possibility of hope and challenged to use our creative powers in reconciliation, but the ultimate decision rests with us.

We know we cannot go back to the same thing. We must begin again or draw further apart, and the choices are more apparent to us now than they were when we first experienced romantic love. Then it seemed that the grace of our sexual drive was so overpowering that we had little choice. God does not directly intervene in our relationship now; rather we experience our sexual attraction as a renewal of the initial invitation to respond to the divine lure to beauty.

When we respond positively to this invitation from our body and the body of our lover—whether this response is immediate and intensely passionate sex or slow and easy sex—we find that sex gets better. The rubber band pulls us back from the edge of disaster and we are reminded of the Bible words, now put to song, "Come back to me, long have I waited for your coming home."

Our sex in beginning again is procreative in the sense that we are starting something new in the midst of a void; we are creating a new bond between us. At this time we sense the need for fertility in our sex, we sense that what takes place here matters to others. Our intercourse becomes aware of its location at the core of a system. Successful marital intimacy reverberates through the family and, to a great extent, determines family happiness. We are generating an environment in which family love can again flourish. Our children, and possibly even our friends, benefit from our new-found joy at falling in love again.

The sexual communication of beginning again is essentially religious because it contains the message that we are loved and that we will survive. Physical, sexual behavior orients us not only to reproduction, but also to certifying our sense of survivability; we will survive the loneliness and the anxieties and the shames that have kept us apart, both in settling down and bottoming out. We are now able to share with our lover the illusory quality of such fracturing devices. Our spouse now knows the worst about us, and he still has a passion for us.

We find that in the shift of consciousness accompanying our sexual play, our beginnings (both as individuals and as lovers) return. In our sex we strip down to our earliest years, taste once again the origins of our sensual life, and piece ourselves together anew. The chaos that surfaced in bottoming out is ordered and our passion erupts without damage.

Whatever way we choose to positively respond to the invitation of our bodies, we find that the conscious work of reconciliation is an intrinsic part of our moving together; it is a difficult, sometimes painful, but always creative process. We have to mine the memory of previous courtings and seductions, as well as the old covenants between us, to find the skills to renew ourselves. The work of reconciliation begins as we come to a fuller insight into where we have gone wrong. We then can ask for forgiveness and in turn hear our spouse ask us for forgiveness.

In the early moments of our coming back together, we feel a wrenching pain as we reenact the damage we have done to ourselves and to our lover. We experience the shame of our now obvious motives, which we once thought were virtuous. In order to prevent the persistence of anger and the development of grudges, we must be explicit about what caused our bottoming out. The process of reconciliation can never succeed if we hid the dimensions of our anger from our spouse and hold even one of our perceived hurts against him.

The practice of repentance and forgiveness is analogous to delicate political negotiations or an intricate dance. As we move through a series of marital cycles, we develop our own language of reconciliation, a series of codes that is unique to us.

Timing of reconciliation messages is very important; both of us have to be ready. If we are asking for forgiveness, we must be patient enough to wait until the worst of our spouse's anger dies down before we can reasonably expect her to respond to our advance. At the same time we have to be persistent in asking her for forgiveness. It's important for both of us that we don't give up.

One colloquium member described how, after a marital quarrel, he asks for forgiveness: he calls his wife on the phone from time to time during the work day. If she answers him with a gruff voice, he knows he must wait a while. He will keep calling at certain intervals until he detects hopeful signs in the tone of her voice.

There is always the danger that in our hurt and anger we will withhold forgiveness beyond the time really necessary to vent our anger, and our spouse might do the same. When we are the injured party, we have the option of continuing to feed the fire of our rage and put off forgiveness. After a certain point our refusal to accept an attempt to reconcile becomes sadistic and punishing. We are refusing the grace of the moment.

Many of us in the colloquium had discovered the usefulness of humor in the process of getting an angry and resentful spouse to "come around." One of our members referred to the "jollying" which works so well for him and his wife. This form of "kidding" in a hopeful manner is particularly useful at certain points for bringing an angry spouse out of his anger. Most of us use it without even stopping to think about it. Somehow it just seems appropriate at certain times (not when our spouse is in her darkest mood) to say, in a gentle way, "Come on. Snap out of it; we have better things to do than mope around like this." As one member stated, "Humor is an old marriage trick, and the sooner we learn it, the better." Jollying or kidding seems to free our desire from the bonds of anger that have hidden our wish to be happy again. If we can make a stern, remote-looking spouse *laugh*, all is not lost. There is hope for us yet!

We also need to be able to receive forgiveness. Sometimes, even after we have asked for our spouse's forgiveness and she has freely bestowed it, we find ourselves unable to trust that she really means it. Perhaps we feel we have wronged her so badly that she cannot possibly mean it when she says she accepts our apology. Or it could be that our initial attempt at reconciliation was so enthusiastically received that we realize we are going to have to begin to change our behavior, and we are not yet ready for that. Not to trust our lover's acceptance of our apology is another refusal of the grace of the moment. We need to remember the myraid times Yahweh forgave Israel. We need to hear anew the message of the Prodigal Son parable. We must come out of our hiding and trust that, even after our miserable behavior, we are a lovable person, important to our spouse. Though this seems unbelievable to us, it is true. When we are able to trust, we begin to grasp, as Karl Rahner says, "the radical depths of God's love." We can do this in our marriage when we trust the love with which our spouse forgives us.

We are challenged, as we engage in the process of reconciliation, to speak correctly about the real issues. Rather than doubt our lover's ability to forgive us, we should recognize that she is ready to hope just when we were ready to give up and had nothing to celebrate. It is amazing that she would forgive us, but not unbelievable. She, like Yahweh inviting Israel to hope in Second Isaiah, speaks with what Brueggemann calls a language of amazement.

She says that no matter what, she will not forsake us. With Yahweh she said, "But my love for you will never leave you and my covenant with you will never be shaken" (Isa. 54:10). And in her amazing forgiveness we are challenged to join with her in expressing the hopes and yearnings denied for so long and suspressed so deeply that we are not even aware of them.

When we are sorting out the problem areas between us, forgiving one another for past weakness and transgressions is not enough. The question we must also face is, "What are we going to do about this?" What will we continue to accept about each other, and what needs to be changed in order to avoid a repeat of the particular transgressions that precipitated the bottoming out?

This is a time for listening and sharing as never before (each time we begin again, we reveal more and more of ourselves to each other). We have to let one another know what we really need and want from each other.

When we speak with the language of amazement, we are free to share our real needs, not just the ones we had thought were appropriate. It is not enough for our spouse to know that we were dissatisfied with certain aspects of our sex life; for any change to occur we have to be able to share with him our fantasies of what we want him to be like as a sexual partner, what we had always dreamed he would do to us, what particular seduction scenes, fondlings, and caresses we want. A major transition occurs when we move from secretly blaming our spouse for not delivering what we want in our fantasy and actually sharing our sexual dreams openly with him. We begin to take responsibility for our own needs. We ask for things we didn't ask for before when, in our shame, we were silent, but privately (and sometimes quite openly) resented our spouse for not knowing.

The sharing of sexual fantasies is both pleasurable and difficult. In the back of our minds we are always asking ourselves if our spouse is going to think we are abnormal, or if he will refuse even to listen to us. It is always harder to tell a spouse what he is doing to excite us (and to ask for things we know will be exciting for us), than it is to tell him what is *not* working. Once we begin to trust, after being forgiven for our part in bottoming out, it becomes easier to share those things that make us feel good, not just the dissatisfactions.

The sharing of the language of perversity (by perversity we mean a celebration of diversity and appreciation of spontaneity and surprise) allows each of us to nurture our sense of survivability—the other hears our secret thoughts and we are still loved. Our intimacy is strengthened and our sense of trust increased. We become like the young child who has no shame about his body, who delights in the wonders he discovers in it, and has no compunction about showing his appreciation of it. And we are amazed. How is it that such good could come out of something so bad (bottoming out)?

At this point we resemble Jacob in his battle with the night visitor (Gen. 32:24-32). He is wounded and changed in the process of the battle, but even in his wounded state he somehow has prevailed. As James Whitehead observes:

> Success in intimacy . . . is rather a matter of wrestling to a new relationship. In this relationship both . . . are altered

and yet both prevail. To prevail is to survive the ambiguous embrace, to know it as an embrace of care, rather than of control.

We have battled through the dark night of bottoming out and both been wounded, yet in the sunrise of beginning again we discover new wonders that make the dark night an empowering experience.

In addition to listening with empathy to each other's fears and fantasies, we now challenge our spouse and are challenged by her. Our spouse's sexual and emotional needs are an invitation to us, and ours are one to her. For example, we may tell our wife that we would especially like to be seduced by an aggressive woman (many men have this fantasy). This revelation of our fantasy is seen as a challenge by her—will she do it for us? She might find the idea of being an aggressive seductress tantalizing, but very new to her—and loaded with negative connotations (i.e., it is not an "appropriate" or "nice" feminine role). We have asked her to create a new role, to reveal a dimension of herself that she is not comfortable with. How can we present our challenge as an invitation, not as a demand? How do we challenge supportively in a marriage? The following tale shows how one man challenged his wife:

> A husband has long had a desire to see his wife wear a particular type of erotic lingerie—the kind that would, in her mind, only be worn by mistresses or prostitutes. He knows if he simply suggests this to her, she will have a difficult time bringing herself to buy it. Since he very much wants his fantasy to come true, he buys her the lingerie and gives it to her as a present. She is overcome with mixed emotions—delight and surprise, embarrassment and fear. (How will she look in it? Will she be able to be the seductress he wants?) He sees that to demand that she try it on immediately would cause her much anxiety. So he waits, letting her know that he wants her to wear it only when she has resolved some of the strong ambivalences she feels about appearing in it. When she finally does work up the

courage, he responds with such delight and pleasure that there is no doubt in her mind that she is irresistible as a seductress.

In this second story, the wife does the challenging:

> A woman enjoys a particular fantasy of being surprised in the middle of the day by her husband. She imagines him coming in to her with an aroused look in his eyes; he takes her by the hand and says, "Come on, let's get out of here!" He drives her to a secluded resort where they have lunch, during which he can barely keep his hands off of her. He then takes her to a sunlit room which he has reserved especially for them, and they make love for the entire afternoon. When the woman reveals her fantasy to her husband, he is at once intrigued, but also feels somewhat uncomfortable about doing something so spontaneous, romantic, and out-of-the-ordinary. He has doubts that he would be able to plan such a wonderful escape. His wife, who realizes she must be a little more concrete about her desires before he can learn to surprise her in the way she wants, describes to him the kind of place she would like to go to, what she would like him to wear, etc. When they do experience the joys of leisurely lunch-and-lovemaking in the afternoon, and the husband observes the delightful effect upon his wife, he gains a new confidence in himself as a lover.

In the first story, the husband knows that both he and his wife have entered marriage with certain limitations in terms of their fears, shames, and negative self-images. He accepts that, but he is open to new possibilities for her and to the development of potential dimensions of her personality that would increase her appeal to him. He tries to make it possible for her to accept his invitation without obstructing her freedom or increasing her fear. He gives her the time she needs.

In the second story, the husband *wants* to escape with his wife, not because he feels obligated to, but because she has told him of a way in which he can be irresistible to her and exert a power to arouse her that he didn't have before. He is open to the possibility that spending an afternoon of lovemaking at a resort may bring delights to both of them that they had not experienced previously.

These stories are models for the paradox of acceptance and challenge in marital intimacy. We all come into marriage with certain equipment (our bodies, our personalities, and our positive and negative feelings about both of these), and we have to know and understand our limits in certain areas. But the role of each of us is to strongly encourage each other—in a nonthreatening way—to discover possibilities that have been hidden beneath our fears and inhibitions. We assume the reality of our limitations and imperfections; we need also to assume the reality of the ever present possibility. We can become the new man/woman, and the process of beginning again in our marriage cycle presents us with an opportunity to explore some of the possibilities of the new person. While finitude is built into creatureliness (we know we can't be the God we want to be in our fantasies), we sin when we give up hope that we can possibly change.

The issues of challenge and change, so obvious as we move through the beginning again period, are undoubtedly two of the most difficult tasks we face on our journey. Yet, when we are successful at these, we, like the husband and wife in the stories, are amazed at the joy we both give and receive. Again, intimacy (with the development of the skills of intimacy) is its own reward.

If our challenge to our spouse is one that will lead to an enrichment of our intimacy, it has to be a challenge to him to be the best he can be. This means that we must be able to "get inside his skin" and know his world from *his* perspective. We have to be particularly adept at listening to him so we know *his* world, know it with our minds, our bodies, and our hearts. Only then can we feel with him and know who he really is. When we are successful at that, it is possible to more effectively evaluate whether what we are asking from him is actually a challenge to *his* possibilities or a challenge based on what *we* want his possibilities to be.

It is helpful, when we are trying to challenge our spouse, to remember Yahweh's words when Moses asks, "What am I to tell them?" (if they ask the name of the God of their fathers). Yahweh replies, according to recent biblical scholars' interpretation of the Hebrew words, "I will be with you forever, but as I am, not as you would have me be" (Exod. 3:13-14). We only have the right to challenge the "who I am" of our spouse. And we will only begin to know the "who I am" when we listen attentively to the other, to his words and to his absence of words, both of which tell us a little bit at a time who he is.

So it is that at this time in marriage we begin the practice of making negotiable demands. We begin to ask our spouse, in a nonthreatening way, for things we would like to see changed, while we remain open to the possibility that she will not be able to respond to our request. We will never be able to fully know "who she is," so we must admit our finitude and be willing to negotiate a solution that might give us less than we had originally wanted. She must be free to say "no" without being made to feel guilty for saying it.

The paradox of intimacy that becomes evident at this point is that of mutuality and identity. How is it that we can share our identities with another and still retain a sense of ourselves? How do we integrate the pull to personal survival and the pull to sexual union so that the harmony of both displays the necessary contrasts inevitably caused by the two pulls? As we move through each cycle on our journey to genuine intimacy (communion of persons), we become more skilled at allowing the contrast between mutuality and identity to be part of the beauty of our intimacy. We learn in the move from bottoming out to beginning again that we can survive some contrasts. We are perhaps hearing a hint of the possibility that the genuine intimacy we seek is one in which the existence of contrasts adds to the beauty of it. Although we were created with the divine image calling us to union, there is no reason to think that the union forces us to give up our identity. If love were to mean union without contrasts, Yahweh would have made us all the same at the start.

As a response to our spouse's attempts to develop the skill to challenge us, we need to consider our own ability to change. What does change represent to us? Why are we so often afraid to consider the possibility of change? What are some of the values of change for us and for our relationship? We need, at this point in our marriage, to come to know ourselves. We find that unless we ask ourselves hard questions about "who I am," we will not be able to share that "who I am" with our spouse. Most of us are afraid of taking stock. We do not want to surrender comfortable habits, even when they are nonproductive. It has taken us years to build up an image of ourselves and we fear the consequences of breaking it down. We tend to grab on to Yahweh's response to Moses and say, "That's right; let me be as I am. Don't try to change me."

We are faced with the challenge here of developing a new self-image that allows for the possibility of growth and change in our lives no matter how old we might be. We are like the man who finds a treasure hidden in the field and the merchant who finds the pearl of great choice (Matt. 13:44-45). We have found a gracious and joyous gift in the rediscovery of the possibility of intimacy with our spouse. But if we want to have that treasure, we must sell all that we have (our comfortable self-image) and reappraise our past views and values. Only then will we be able to buy, that is, give an empowering response to the challenge brought on by the opportunities of beginning again. If we see our spouse as fundamentally good and worthy of our trust, if we are able to perceive that the opportunity of our renewed relationship is another manifestation of God's gracious gift to us, we find that our life is being transformed from old to new.

We discover in this process of beginning again that the throes of intimacy are inevitably the throes of transformation. And where this transformation from isolation to communion (assisted by our ability to put on a new person) is happening, the God of transformation is present. As our life is transformed from the old to the new, God and love are being reborn.

We are like Jacob. We were not only wounded in the dark night of bottoming out, but we also find that we were changed. We are, if we are willing to respond to the grace of beginning again, able to give up something of ourselves without feeling that we have lost much of value in the process. As we disclose and reveal ourselves to our spouse, we find we have been returned to the Promised Land, we have been raised with Jesus, we are the disciples with Jesus in our midst after the Resurrection. We are Paul and the Corinthians after they have refound each other in the shared story of their beginnings. We are ready to enter into a new covenant with our spouse.

We begin to speak with the language of covenant, which is a language about our faithfulness to each other. We find ourselves in Second Isaiah with words of hope and praise. We are comforted, and our comfort is not just because we have a nice feeling. It grows out of the deep conviction that we have overthrown the powers of fatigue that kept us apart. It is time for us to sing a new song (Ps. 98).

When we enter the light of the new morning, we are in the midst of festival time. We want to shout with joy at our newfound rebirth. We find that the despair of the night has been reversed and with our spouse we bring to the present the wonder of falling in love. We have given birth to a new love, and with our new covenant we are able to confront our despair and create a forward movement on the spiral of marital intimacy.

What began as an intimidating experience, as threat and injury, is transformed mysteriously into growth. In this experience we have learned the nuances and skills of surviving. At the end of the struggles we are at a new beginning, the beginning of a new covenant, full of hope and promise.

BEGINNING AGAIN

We shall not cease from exploration
and the end of all our exploring
will be to arrive where we started
and know the place for the first time.
T.S. Eliot,   *Little Gidding*

Conclusion

We arrive at the end of our love story only to find that we are at the beginning of a new cycle on our spiral of marital intimacy. We have completed one cycle and have been enriched by our discovery of the transcendent and the tragic possibilities in our intimacy—the transcendent going out of ourselves in falling in love and beginning again; the tragic awareness of our sin in settling down and bottoming out. We also find that the second telling of our love story will probably be much better than the first. We have become more adept in our sexual intimacy; the rubber band is stronger and we should be better lovers.

As we begin another cycle of marital intimacy, we move a bit closer to genuine intimacy (communion of persons), the divine lure to beauty for humans with the divine image imprinted in our bodies from the moment of our creation. We will undoubtedly experience this cycle again and again—sometimes with greater tragedy, other times with the enrichment of the transcendent. We now know that the quest for genuine intimacy is a lifelong quest. We cannot settle for apparent harmony at any time since, once we have achieved a level of harmony and developed a pattern of relating, the routine causes the intimacy to wane. We continually need to move on to a higher level of intimacy.

Though it is not good for man—male and female—to be alone, we see that the pull to personal survival (to be alone) will constantly plague us as we continue our intimacy journey. The better equipped we are with an imagination that tells us to follow the lure to beauty, the more apt we are not to stay frozen too long in periods of false harmony or disharmony.

CONCLUSION

We realize as we review the key moments in our plot that our love story is a challenge to those of us who take the journey of marital intimacy and to the Catholic Christian community who look to our journey for a sign of the union of Christ and the church.

Since the colloquium not only liked to think big, but also to give advice, we are following up our vision (thinking big) with some conclusions (giving advice) that flow from the vision. Our conclusions pertain to three groups: those taking the marital intimacy journey, the local church community which ministers to married people, and the wider church community which has a responsibility to proclaim a vision for all. We want to reiterate, at this point, that our vision and, therefore, our conclusions speak of possibilities, not of obligations. We have not devised a "how to" for happier marriages; rather we have imagined a vision of what is possible in a marriage. Making this possibility a reality in our lives means adapting it to our own situation. Our conclusions are guidelines that might be helpful for our adaptation.

The vision of marital intimacy discovered through a correlation of life and faith challenges married people to solicit our own potential as we seek to grow in intimacy. We are encouraged to assume *responsibility* for growth in intimacy by *responding* to the gift of sexuality bestowed on us by God. Some suggestions which should assist us as we journey through the cycles are:

1. We shouldn't listen to prophets of gloom. Some say we shouldn't expect to continue to grow in our marriage; most marriages are routine and rather dull and boring; we shouldn't expect more; we should be content with what we have. Then there are those who believe we can't grow in intimacy in one marriage; we should feel free to get out when the growing stops and continue our journey with someone else; it isn't reasonable to expect that we should be held to a commitment.

Both of these represent false prophecies, untrue to the human sexual drive for union and untrue to the giftedness of

CONCLUSION

our sexuality. We can become lovers if we are willing to embrace both the tragic and the transcendent and integrate them on our journey.

2. We should develop our romantic—and religious—imagination. Let's think of our marriage as a love story. How would we write that story? We shouldn't think for a minute that *our* marriage would never make a good love story. The divine plan is that all marriages should be love stories. It's up to us to decide whether we want to go along with the plan. Yahweh wrote the basic love story with the creation of the first humans. Our task is to write the script for our presentation of the story. We also are the producers and directors; we must be prepared for a divine critique of how well we have interpreted the original story.

3. We should celebrate our sexual intimacy. That was why we were created male and female. The pull for personal survival plus bad attitudes and habits developed prior to marriage can interfere with our ability to appreciate our sexuality. If we are unable to overcome these attitudes and habits, we should get help. Seeking assistance in increasing our skills as sexual lovers is a positive response to the grace of our sexuality. It moves us out of the shame we use to isolate ourselves from our beloved. We need to work together to help each other break down barriers.

We have to acknowledge our ignorance about certain facets of sexual intimacy. Only then will we be able to avoid the dilemma of the couple who went to a sex therapy clinic seeking help for the husband's impotency. He was only interested in having sexual relations three times a week. Having relied on tales of sexual powers picked up along the way, this poor couple thought he had a physical problem. We must seek out knowledgeable sources when we have a question.

And if we still have problems, we should consider the option of sex therapy. Again, we should be careful about where we seek such help. Generally a good starting point is a clinic attached to a respected university hospital or a reputable community hospital that has board-certified psychiatrists who are either doing the therapy or supervising it.

4. We should develop human relation skills. These are mandatory if we hope to be successful in our journey. If we don't have them, we ought to develop them. If we do have them, we probably need to improve on them. We need to practice self-disclosure, empathy, challenge, reconciliation. We need to acknowledge our vulnerability so we can be trusting. We need to learn how to express anger in a positive way. If we become skilled at these, we will probably be better lovers. What a waste to pretend we can't. Again here, if we need professional help to rid us of the barriers making it impossible for us to practice these skills, we should seek it. The reward of intimacy is too great to pass up.

5. We should pay more attention to what is going on in our story and in the story of our religious tradition. There are so many diversions to our hopeful vision of marriage that we need to dialogue continually with the richness of our religious tradition. We need to keep ourselves open to the possibilities of grace within our intimacy. To do this we have to listen to what is going on in our marriage. We need to reflect on both the marriage and the tradition. We need sacred time and sacred space together with our spouse so we will be able to mine the riches of our marriage and our tradition. Though our religious stories and symbols are not substitutes for techniques of self-knowledge, communication, and understanding the psyche, there is a vision of affection, candor, and love in these stories. They stress that union is the sole way to happiness and peace and that selflessness is the way to salvation. Happiness, we find in the New Testament, includes the love of our neighbor (spouse).

6. We should develop our own language of grief. We need to learn how to express our feeling of grief at the discovery of our sinful rejection of our spouse in order to begin the journey from Good Friday to Easter.

7. We should develop our own language of reconciliation.

CONCLUSION

We need to be people who know how to ask for, give, and receive forgiveness. We need to learn how to repair what we have done when we have sinned against each other.

8. We should develop our own language of amazement. We need to learn how to celebrate, be perverse, develop rituals which bring our beginning back to us—sexual rituals and other relational rituals.

Those of us who have embarked on the journey of marital intimacy realize that we need all the help we can get if we are to be successful in reaching our goal. Since our vision of marital intimacy is based on our Catholic Christian tradition, it is only natural that we would look for support from our religious community. So it is that we turn to a consideration of the way in which a local church supports its members as they struggle to implement the suggestions which flow from our vision. Local churches support our journey when they:

1. Understand the importance of a spirituality of marital intimacy. Local church leaders—clerical, religious, and lay—need to recognize the importance of inspiration for those of us on the journey of marital intimacy. When they listen to our experiences and present us with images, symbols, and stories from our faith tradition, they assist us in our quest.

2. Develop liturgies and homilies which incorporate the language of grief, the language of reconciliation, and the language of amazement in a celebration of human sexuality and marital intimacy. We should not participate in Sunday after Sunday of liturgies while in the midst of bottoming out and never hear a challenge to respond to the wonder of our sexuality.

3. Offer programs—retreats, talks, adult education, marriage education—which help us mine the richness of our marital intimacy and of our religious tradition. We think improving our human relations skills and our understanding of our sexuality are ways in which we learn how to respond to the challenge to love imprinted on us; learning to do this is

a religious task and we should do it in our religious community.

Although *some* people will benefit from *some* premarital education, the best marriage education begins with the small baby. Opportunities to develop our human relations and religious skills, especially during the crucial periods of settling down, bottoming out, and beginning again, will assist us as we seek to educate our babies and reeducate ourselves.

4. Coordinate a resource center where we can seek advice about the best professional help. A periodic evaluation of the best help in sex therapy and marital and family therapy—made available to all the members of the community—provides an opportunity for us to respond to grace when we most need it.

5. Encourage support groups within the religious community. The vision of marriage imagined from a correlation of life and faith requires a sharing with those who have the same faith perspective. Embracing the tragic possibilities of marriage and going outside of ourselves in response to the transcendent is not always an easy task. Nor is it one which receives enthusiastic support from the secular community. If we are to wax with our vision, rather than continually wane, we need to share this vision with others; we need to have our interpretation of it reinforced by others.

Finally, our journey of marital intimacy will flourish in a wider church community which loudly proclaims a positive vision of marital intimacy. We see this positive vision emanating from a variety of sources: the pope, synods, national conferences of bishops, clergy and other pastoral leaders, scholars in the social sciences and theology and the biological sciences, and Catholic universities. The wider church community encourages the quest for marital intimacy when:

1. Papal statements celebrate marital intimacy using the language of the Creation story, the Song of Songs, Jerimiah,

CONCLUSION

Second Isaiah, the Incarnation, Good Friday, and Easter. These statements should offer encouragement and support for the journey and not deal with a static ideal, which to most of us comes across as boring and dull. Religious language for the journey should be a language of grief, reconciliation, and amazement, not a language of rules. Codes, when needed, should be related to wonder at a God who has created us to love.

2. Papal statements on marital intimacy reflect a familiarity with the experience of married life. Abstract theological discourses are quite appropriate (and even necessary) for setting forth the basis for marital intimacy, but such discourses should also be rooted in an appreciation of the journey we are on. Theological discourses should then be translated into a language which the nontheologian will understand. Otherwise we miss the inspiration of these messages.

Such statements will be most effective when they demonstrate an understanding of *our* experience of marriage—not necessarily our individual story, but at least the story of people in our situation in life, whatever it might be.

3. Synods meet to discover what is the best correlation of life and faith at this time in human history. Participation in these synods should be open to those who are concerned with the issues in their daily lives, at least in some advisory capacity. Synod statements on marital intimacy need input from women. Wives have a crucial role to play in the quest for marital intimacy and they should critically reflect on this and express their views.

4. National conferences of bishops articulate a vision of marital intimacy for the people they serve. We are not so naive as to believe that marital intimacy is only a possibility for people in our advanced technological and affluent society. We believe that there is much to be learned from other experiences of intimacy that would be incorporated in the vision formulated by various conferences. In addition, the past habit of speaking out on human sexuality without

any consideration of the journey of marital intimacy has led married people all over the world to think the church is not interested in inspiring us in the area of marital intimacy. National conferences which speak to the needs of their particular countries would support the intimacy journey of their own people. They would also be better equipped to contribute to a vision of marriage for the universal church.

5. Clergy (pope, cardinals, bishops, pastors, associate pastors, deacons) and other pastoral leaders are people who demonstrate a capacity for intimacy in their own lives. When pastoral leaders, by their own lifestyles, proclaim a vision of people created to be lovers, they are living proof of God's plan. Clergy who love their people, whoever those people are, are continuing the program begun by Yahweh and practiced by Jesus.

6. Catholic scholars are dedicated to the study of the possibility of marital intimacy. The hierarchy of the church cannot intuit what the problems and challenges of sexual intimacy are for a particular people. Scholars need to research the issues and supply the hierarchy with the results of their work. (It is important that the hierarchy take some intiative and request and fund such research.) Areas of research which contribute vital information to a vision of intimacy include the social sciences, theology, and those areas of the biological sciences that study human sexuality.

7. Catholic universities are willing to dedicate a portion of their resources to the study of the issues pertinent to human intimacy. Bringing together the resources of theologians and other scientists interested in marital intimacy in one place would insure a public recognition of the Catholic Christian interest in this topic.

Our vision of marital intimacy as a love story leads us to call for married people, the local church, and the universal church to focus their resources on this issue. If private and public imagination are able to imagine the impossible and work toward implementing what is imagined, men and

CONCLUSION

women will be encouraged to discover the meaning of their existence in their quest for marital intimacy. In turn, married people who are lovers will begin to reveal the meaning of love to others.

God created us with the divine image imprinted on our bodies so we might become lovers and discover in our love the essence of life. When we respond to the divine plan, we widely proclaim the glory of God. We become lovers so all can see the wonders of the divine. Intimacy is its own reward for us and for our God.

Working Papers Prepared for Various Sessions of the Colloquium

The Experience of Intimacy

"Intimacy and Conflict: A Personal Reflection"
Marilyn and Kevin Ryan

"Self-Concept and Marriage"
Marilyn and Kevin Ryan

"Problems in Intimacy: Perspectives from Sex Therapy"
Daniel and Joan Anzia

"Shame and Perversity: Physical Sexuality and Religion in the Life Cycle"
William McCready

"Sex, Intimacy, and Family Systems Theory"
John Durburg

"Sex and Marriage: For Pre-Marriage and Post-Marriage Consideration"
Kevin and Marilyn Ryan

The Social Context

"Numbering Our Days Aright: Human Longevity and the Problem of Intimacy"
Teresa Sullivan

"The Sacred Center: Sexuality, Religion, and Fertility in Families"
John Kotre

"Religion and the Life Cycle"
William McCready

"Intimacy in Catholic Family Life: An Empirical Investigation"
William McCready

"The Origins of Religious Persistence: Sexual Identity and Religious Socialization"
William and Nancy McCready

Theological Reflections on Intimacy

"A Biblical Model of Human Intimacy: The Song of Songs"
Roland E. Murphy

"Intimacy and the New Testament"
John Kilgallen

"A Theological Perspective on Human Relations Skills and Family Intimacy"
John Shea

"Growing in Human Intimacy and the Parables"
Bruno V. Manno

"Intimacy and Marriage: Continuing the Mystery of Christ and the Church"
Mary G. Durkin

"The Catholic Model of Caritas: Self-Transcendence and Transformation"
David Tracy

Secondary Sources Used for Some Key Themes in the Story

Brueggemann, Walter. *The Prophetic Imagination.* Philadelphia: Fortress Press, 1978. Especially rich in ideas for bottoming out and beginning again.

Cobb, John. *A Christian Natural Theology.* Philadelphia: Westminster, 1965, pp. 92-135. Discussion of the process view of the divine lure to beauty and the cycle of harmony and disharmony.

Whitehead, James. *Christian Life Patterns: Psychological Tasks and Religious Invitation in Adult Life.* New York: Doubleday, 1979, ch. 4. Material on Jacob.